S0-BWQ-350

Treating Neck Problems the Natural Way

GOODBYE PAIN IN THE NECK

Dr. S.S. Neel with Sandra C. Craig

Illustrated by Jeff Buchwitz

PUBLISHER
HEALTH CHALLENGES TODAY INC.
1990

"Those who do not feel pain seldom think that it is felt."
SAMUEL JOHNSON

Copyright ©1990
    Sarbjit Singh Neel

    No part of this book may be reproduced or transmitted in any form by any means, electronic or mechanical, including photocopying and recording, or by any information storage or retrieval system without written permission from the authors, except for brief passages quoted in a review.

Canadian Cataloguing in Publication Data
    Neel, Sarbjit Singh, 1958 - Treating Neck Problems the Natural Way: Goodbye Pain in the Neck
    ISBN 0-9694691-0-1
    1. Neck pain. 2. Neck pain – Treatment. 3. Whiplash injuries – Chiropractic treatment.
I. Craig, Sandra. C. II. Health Challenges Today (Delta, B.C.). III. Title RZ265.N4N43 1990
617.5'306 C90-091465-3

Cartoon illustrations by: Jeff Buchwitz

Cover by: Reinhard Derreth Graphics Ltd.
Typesetting by: The Typeworks
Printed and bound in Canada by: Hignell Printing Limited

Published by:
Health Challenges Today Inc.
11133 Prospect Drive Delta, B.C. Canada V4E 2R4
Telephone: (604) 599-8688
FAX: (604) 599-5523

For information:
Dr. S.S. Neel
Scott – 72 Professional Offices
#216-7313 – 120th Street
Delta, British Columbia, Canada
V4C 6P5
Telephone: (604) 599-8699
FAX: (604) 599-5523

DEDICATED TO OUR
FAMILIES, FRIENDS AND PATIENTS

IF YOU HAVE A NECK...
THIS BOOK IS FOR YOU

This book is designed for individuals with **healthy necks** who want to keep them that way, and for those with **painful necks** who want relief from suffering and to join the **healthy!**

Specific therapeutic exercises are provided in each chapter. They will help you to strengthen your neck, improve your posture and the alignment of your spine, and decrease the stress and pain in your neck – thus allowing you to enjoy work and play at your maximum potential.

Exercises to be incorporated in your daily routine for a healthy and flexible neck are discussed in **Exercises for a Healthy Neck** (chapter 32).

This book is not intended to replace the care provided by your health professional. Use your discretion in applying the recommendations outlined in this book.

NOTE: EXERCISES ARE MOST BENEFICIAL WHEN UNDERTAKEN IN CONJUNCTION WITH THE TREATMENT PROVIDED BY YOUR HEALTH CARE PRACTITIONER.

ABOUT THE AUTHORS

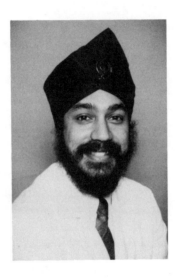

Dr. Sarbjit (Sarj) Singh Neel, D.C. was born in East Africa. He graduated from McNair Senior Secondary School in Richmond, British Columbia and took pre-medical studies at the University of British Columbia. In 1982 Dr. Neel graduated from Western States Chiropractic College in Portland, Oregon. He is a past member of the B.C. Track and Field Team, a recipient of many awards and medals for outstanding achievement in sprinting events, and was responsible for organizing the First Fitness Festival for Richmond's Centennial year. Since 1983 Dr. Neel has been in private practise and has a specific interest in Whiplash Injury. He is a noted writer on Whiplash Injury and Soft Tissue Trauma as well as an internationally recognized expert and lecturer on these subjects. For the past three years Dr. Neel has coordinated the Annual International Multi-Disciplinary Symposium on Spinal Trauma and Whiplash Injury, the first of its kind in North America, which has attracted world-renowned expert speakers. Apart from health care Sarj is an accomplished musician and has produced and released with his wife, Kamaljit (Kami) an uptempo traditional music tape called SHAWA. Sarj and Kami live in Sunshine Hills, Delta, British Columbia.

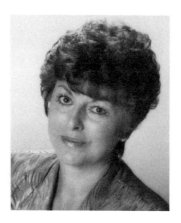

Sandra C. Craig was born in England and educated in Canada. She has been a business consultant and a human resources recruitment specialist for over 20 years. Mrs. Craig has written numerous articles and reports on health issues and in 1983 published *Strong Medicine*, an incisive overview of the health care delivery system in British Columbia. Mrs. Craig has been a popular guest on several radio and television shows about consumer health issues and has hosted her own television program, **It's Your Health**. She has also lectured at universities and community health centres as a consumer advocate of patients' rights. Sandra resides in a wilderness home on Fromme Mountain in North Vancouver, British Columbia with her husband David and son Dayn.

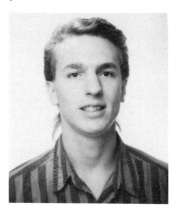

Jeff Buchwitz was born in 1971, in Vancouver, British Columbia. A graduate of Seaquam Secondary School (North Delta, B.C.), he is presently studying graphic design at Kwantlen College. Like his father, Jeff is an excellent water-colour artist. Jeff resides in Delta with his parents, a brother and a sister.

TABLE OF CONTENTS

INTRODUCTION   1
1. FUNCTIONAL ANATOMY OF THE NECK   3
2. DO YOU HAVE GOOD NECK POSTURE?   6
3. HOW WELL DOES YOUR NECK MOVE?   10
4. BODY LANGUAGE: WHAT IS PAIN?   14
5. WHIPLASH: A MODERN-DAY CURSE   16
6. WHIPLASH – ITS SYMPTOMS: "THE MANY FACES OF EVE" SYNDROME   19
7. WHIPLASH: FACTORS INFLUENCING ITS EXTENT AND SEVERITY   22
8. YOUR WHIPLASH CLAIM: INSURANCE, ADJUSTERS AND YOU   24
9. THE WHEN AND WHERE OF WHIPLASH OCCURRENCE   27
10. WHIPLASH: WERE YOUR HEAD AND NECK ROTATED?   28
11. WHIPLASH – HEAD RESTRAINTS: ARE YOURS ADJUSTED CORRECTLY?   31
12. "OH, MY SPLITTING HEADACHE!"   33
13. WHIPLASH – NECK COLLARS: DO THEY HELP?   38
14. X-RAYS: RADIOGRAPHIC EXAMINATION   41
15. THE OSTEOARTHRITIC OR DEGENERATIVE NECK   44
16. TRIGGER POINTS: WHAT ARE THEY AND HOW DO THEY INFLUENCE PAIN?   48
17. RADICULOPATHY: NERVE ROOT DAMAGE AND REFERRED PAIN   51
18. HYPERMOBILITY: ARE YOU A GRINDER?   54
19. PROGNOSIS: HOW WELL WILL I BE?   58
20. PILLOW TALK: CHOOSING A NECK PILLOW   60
21. SHOULD YOU APPLY COLD OR HEAT?   63
22. NECK POSTURE AND JAW PAIN: "CHEWING THE FAT" CAN BE PAINFUL   66
23. WRY NECK: ACUTE SPASMODIC TORTICOLLIS   68
24. STRESS, TENSION, EMOTIONAL PROBLEMS AND NECK PAIN   70
25. OCCUPATIONAL PAIN TRIGGERS   73
26. WHAT ARE YOU WEARING AROUND YOUR NECK?   77
27. CHILDBIRTH AND THE CHILD'S NECK   79

28. SPORTS INJURIES: ARE YOU A HEAD BANGER?   81
29. SEX AND THE NECK   83
30. THE IMPORTANCE OF FEEDING YOUR NECK TISSUES WELL   85
31. CHOOSING A PRACTITIONER   87
32. EXERCISES FOR A HEALTHY NECK   88
33. SMASHING EXCUSES   96
34. GOODBYE PAIN IN THE NECK   98
35. ADDITIONAL SUGGESTED READING ON
    NECK AND WHIPLASH INJURIES   100

FOREWORD

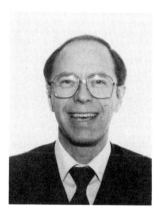

Neck pain can permeate deep into every pore of our body, right into our soul. To add insult to injury, there are many shortcomings on the part of the health professions – we have failed to bring to the neck sufferer the necessary information upon which he or she can base an informed opinion about his or her pain.

Believe me, it is the sufferer's pain and nobody else's. We can use words to describe pain, but we can't pick it up and show it around, nor can we cut it out. There are dramatic injuries that cause obvious damage to neck structures, and the health professions have described these well; but the common neck pain is not dramatic and is poorly described. The average person knows little about the neck, but everyone has one, and should know more.

It all goes back to mother nature; she placed too large a brain, in too large a head, on too large an ego, with too small a neck. Only in science fiction do you see such strange creatures with large globular knobs sticking out on flimsy stalks. We stick our necks out too often, and suffer the consequences. We can't redo the design of the neck, but we can make what we have stronger and sturdier through exercise.

Scientific studies on soft tissue sprains and strains have shown that early intervention with exercise is essential for the proper repair of injuries. In this regard, we cannot ignore the neck by caging it into a collar; that will only lead to disuse atrophy of the neck muscles, thinning of the ligament supports, breakdown of the joints and degeneration of the discs. Regardless of how you look at it, if you don't use your neck, you'll lose it.

Recently it has been said about low back pain that doctors only send their patients to bed if they don't like them. Bed rest is bad for the back. Now we should add: "Only put someone in a neck collar if you want to make them worse." Once you start down the road with a weak neck, it's hard to return – unless you put in the effort.

The biggest problem with necks is not what you do that is wrong, but what you don't do. It's easy to have poor posture. But failure to correct the posture through exercise is the worst of all evils. Where is that little voice inside that says: "Stand up straight, shoulders back, chin in, chest out, keep fit"? We have to constantly remind ourselves of the good things in life. If you have a neck that aches, look after it – it's the only one you've got. There is no warranty, and it can't be returned.

Dr. Sarbjit Neel, D.C., has put together a useful resource book that deals with common neck problems and some simple methods people can use to help themselves and their necks. Essentially he is giving neck sufferers enough information to make informed decisions about how they can look after themselves. He encourages you to take an active role in treating yourself. Don't passively rely on others to do it to you – you must rely on yourself. This is a funny book about a very serious subject, and has important messages for anyone with a "pain in the neck."

Murray E. Allen, M.D.
Associate Professor
School of Kinesiology
Director: Back Centre
Simon Fraser University
Burnaby, B.C. Canada

INTRODUCTION

As a Doctor of Chiropractic I have treated thousands of patients who suffer from minor to severe neck and back pain that make their lives less than sweet.

Simple everyday tasks such as bending over to pick a flower, tend a fragrant garden, retrieve a found "lucky" penny from the ground, or tie a shoelace, or, with the toss of a head, yelling a happy goodbye all become less spontaneous as the body quickly registers the distress such tasks engender. As these actions are triggered, the brain goes into red alert. In less than a microsecond the brain forewarns the body, saying in essence, "forget it, don't do it, you'll feel pain, so back off!" The flower therefore remains unpicked, the fragrant garden becomes tangled – the "country" gardener evolves into the grumpy complainer, and the penny is dismissed as not worth the effort to pick it up. It remains silently on the ground, beckoning a promise of "luck for the day" to the person ready to exert the requisite bend-'n- stretch moves to claim it. The happy over-the-shoulder goodbye remains a thought – not an action. Such is the nature of neck and back pain.

There are many causes of neck and back pain:
- postural changes
- occupational positions
- sports injuries
- traumatic injuries, such as Whiplash

Many of my patients suffer with low back pain as a result of work-related injuries or physical on-the-job stress, as in the case of a shipper/receiver who loads and unloads heavy parcels all day. However, most of my patients who experience neck pain are victims of a Whiplash syndrome.

Unlike those who suffer on-the-job or occupational injury, the Whiplash patient often experiences an insidious "double whammy."

The age-old maxim "seeing is believing" confronts the Whiplash victim at every turn. For example, a broken arm or leg in a cast generates immediate sympathy, understanding and support from friends, relatives, co-workers and the public at large. Even the cast seems to take on a life of its own, becoming a "cause célèbre" with personalized wishes, etchings and humorous anecdotes to brighten up the owner's day. All of this validates the patient's injuries, outlines that the collective consciousness understands – and has sympathy for – the dilemma, particularly if the patient is a golfer who can no longer brag of a "5" handicap!

By contrast, patients experiencing the effects of the "invisible" Whiplash injury are often perceived to be adding "a little dressing to the salad" whenever they wince in pain or complain about a task they cannot fulfill, such as lifting an object or shifting heavy articles.

The patients' "constipated" stiffened walk, poker-straight neck and grimaced face may be the only outward signs of distress visible to the questioning eyes of their detractors. "If it can't be seen, then it isn't there," is the unspoken message, and at times the vocalized critique, emanating from the self-righteous to the sufferer. They are convinced the victim is hamming it up better than Porky the Pig to obtain a bogus insurance settlement, to malinger at work, to dispense with unwanted social commitments or simply to shirk his or her duties. Ironically, the Whiplash patients' pain in the neck makes **them** a pain to others!

However, as a fellow traveller on the road to recovery from Whiplash injury, I can sympathize with the suffering I have seen and treated, which is often caused by internal factors (not recognized by the casual observer) such as spinal misalignments, hairline fractures, torn muscle/ligament tissues and/or traumatized osteoarthritic disc lesions.

The physical and psychological hoops experienced by my patients, combined with the these people's commitment to getting better, have been the inspiration for this book.

Together we will explore a better understanding of how the neck works and what happens when it malfunctions.

At the end of each section I have included exercises for both the treatment and the prevention of neck injuries. These are to be used in conjunction with the care provided by your health practitioner.

Let's act now – and heal the **PAIN IN YOUR NECK!**

1

Functional Anatomy of the Neck

*"Knowledge is of two kinds. We know a
subject ourselves, or we know where we can
find information upon it."*
SAMUEL JOHNSON

We all take our necks for granted – and why not? They've simply always been there! Only episodes of pain or injury draw our attention to just how they function or don't.

As with any delicate mechanism, whether it's our neck or the intricate workings of an antique pocket watch, it helps our appreciation of its value if we understand how vulnerable it is when poorly maintained. And like the antique pocket watch, the neck is a paradox. It is fragile, but incredibly strong and supportive provided it is given the care required to function at full capacity.

The neck is an amazing structure. Its design specifications as provided by nature make the most advanced engineering and scientific wonders of the 20th century, such as computer technology, seem like child's play by comparison. It houses major **arteries** that feed blood and oxygen into the head and brain, the **larynx** (which allows us to breathe), the **pharynx** (responsible for our swallowing mechanism), and thousands of other interconnected blood and nerve vessels. Its primary function, however, is to protect the **spinal cord** (the nerve centre for the body).

Did you know that as you read this book your neck is employing **30** or more muscles to support an average head weight of about **10-12 pounds**? It will perform this task for the rest of your life, barring any injury.

The neck is comprised of seven bony structures known as the **vertebrae**. The vertebrae are connected to an intricate pattern of ligaments and muscles called **soft tissues.** Soft tissues act like a girdle provided by nature, crisscrossing the neck, giving maximum support to its weakest part, known medically as the **atlanto-occipital** region, located at the base of the skull. The vertebrae are separated by a gelatinous material called a **disc.**

Our discs serve more than one function. They act as shock absorbers, so that when we jump or fall they cushion the impact much like the "shocks" of a car. When "shocks" are well maintained and the car hits a bump, you barely feel it – the motion is smooth, free-flowing and effortless. Likewise with healthy discs – they allow freedom of movement to bend, twist, rotate and extend our bodies. Discs also contribute to the overall height of the vertebral column, contributing to one third of the overall length of our spine.

Could you be getting shorter as the day gets longer? Absolutely! This interesting phenomenon results from gravitational forces "squeezing" and compressing naturally occurring fluids out of our discs. This may result in a loss of from ½" to ¾" by the end of the day. Resting at night regenerates the equilibrium of fluids, and restores the disc spaces to their normal height.

Unlike a car's shock absorbers, once our discs are damaged they cannot be replaced. However, they may be partially repaired through surgical intervention, or, if the damage is severe, partially removed. Removal of a disc will result in loss of overall height and reduced movement of the neck.

The **neck** is the most mobile portion of the spine. More than **50 percent** of the rotation motion of the head occurs due to the movement of the first two vertebrae of the neck, called the **atlas** and **axis.**

Have you ever wondered, as you view a glorious sunset, admire an attractive individual walking in front of you, or catch a glimpse of a flashy car racing down the highway, what keeps your eyes focussed straight ahead, parallel to the ground? You probably haven't given it a second thought! But if it weren't for your neck, and specifically the atlas and axis vertebrae acting as precise levers to stabilize your head, such activities would be impossible.

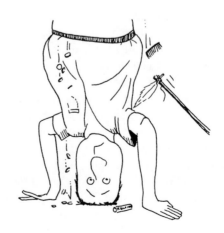

Our necks allow us the freedom to nod, to pull our chins toward our chests, to turn quickly to look over our left or right shoulder (particularly important when approaching a busy intersection), or to move our heads to the left and right when saying "no" to drinks before driving home. We use our necks to look up at the stars, to turn and watch our companion looking up at the stars, and to reach over to plant a kiss on our companion as he or she looks up at the stars! The neck will even support our body weight during a head stand.

Several muscles located in the upper back and in the skull control the movement and position of the neck. In a complementary way, many nerves that control the motor and sensory functions of the arm, upper back and head muscles originate from the neck region. They cause an unusual interaction of pain "referral." For example, injury to the soft tissues or trauma to the discs in the neck may "distress" a nerve, and in turn "refer" or "direct" the pain to another area of the body, such as the hand or the head.

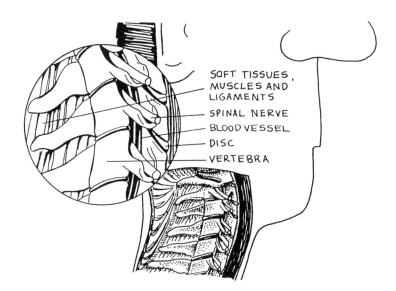

SOFT TISSUES, MUSCLES AND LIGAMENTS

SPINAL NERVE

BLOOD VESSEL

DISC

VERTEBRA

Blood vessels, such as arteries, veins and **lymphatic vessels** (the filtering immune system), regulate the supply of needed oxygen to the neck tissues. Any injury to the neck will affect the normal functioning of these vessels. Tissue damage will result in a decrease in the supply of oxygenated blood. Lack of oxygen in tissues causes pain and dysfunction such as stiffness and loss of mobility.

As we can surmise, a healthy neck is essential to the ability to perform normal, everyday tasks that we otherwise take for granted.

2

Do You Have Good Neck Posture?

"The body follows the head."

The posture of your neck will determine the position in which you hold your head. Many of these stances are developed during adolescence. For example, if you were extremely tall during high school, you probably looked down at your peers and were hunched over. On the other hand, if you were extremely short, you likely developed the habit of extending your neck backward as you looked up. Over time your body will become adapted to these postures. Under such circumstances the slightest trauma to the neck will result in **acute**, or short and severe, symptoms flaring up.

To have ideal posture (looking at the head from the front) both the eyes and ears should be parallel to the ground and level with each other. Likewise, the shoulders should be at the same level. From the side profile (as illustrated below) the person is standing in a relaxed posture. The gravitational or perpendicular line drawn from the centre of the ear falls through the centre portion of the shoulder.

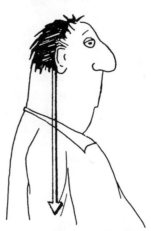

Clinically, practitioners notice that most patients stand with their heads thrust forward. If you are an individual who, like an ostrich, carries the head forward with your chin slightly extended, you will experience a great deal of muscle tension, tightness and fatigue at the base of the neck and the top of the upper back. Why do the muscles hurt in this region?

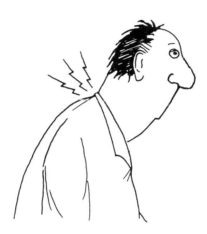

To answer that question, let us envision that you are asked to hold a **10-pound weight** with your arms extended forward. After a short while, the muscles employed to support this weight will become fatigued, and pain will set in throughout the arms and neck. But, if you take the same weight and brace it tightly to your body so that minimal or zero muscle effort is required, you could easily hold this weight for hours.

Similarly, if you have bad posture, the centre of gravity of your head shifts away from your neck and body. Your poor posture stresses the neck muscles, causing the muscles to work harder and burn more energy **just to hold your head up all day!**

If you have a tendency to walk with your shoulders hunched forward, during episodes of physical and mental stress this misaligned stance worsens and your head slouches forward, causing undue stress on the neck.

Remember the three "**P's**":   PRACTISE
PERFECT
POSTURE

TREATMENT AND PREVENTION:

To stengthen the neck's integrity, practise the following exercises:

EXERCISE 1

- Stand in front of a mirror and gently draw or retract your chin backward into your neck.
- Hold this contraction for 5 seconds and repeat 10 times.

This exercise can easily be done in a sitting position while you are at home or work.

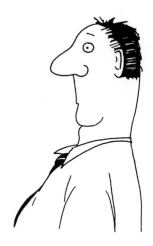

EXERCISE 2

- Lie on a carpet or mat with a pillow under your chest, and your face aligned with the centre of the body (as illustrated).
- Begin by placing both your arms beside you with your palms facing upwards.
- Slowly draw both your shoulder blades toward the centre of your back.
- At the same time, gently lift your face from the ground and retract your chin backward into your neck. Keep the head level with the shoulder blades.
- When the shoulder blades are drawn closely together and the chin is retracted, hold the contraction for 5 seconds. Repeat 10 times.
- Do this exercise twice daily.

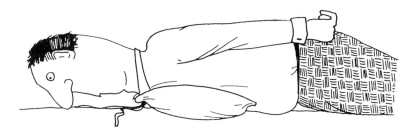

3

How Well Does Your Neck Move?

"Never too old to learn, never too late to turn."

The design of the cervical vertbrae should allow the neck to move in several directions without pain and stiffness. Flexibility and the **range of motion** will vary with age, the natural formation of the bones and, of course, the extent of injury or damage to underlying tissues. For example, a gymnast or a ballerina may have disciplined or conditioned his or her body to move beyond the optimum **average** motion.

To establish how well your neck joints move, let us go through all the motions of the average neck with normal flexibility.

If you experience any sharp pain or dizziness – STOP. Do not push yourself or go any further.

FLEXION or **NODDING TEST**

- Stand straight, shoulders back, with your eyes level.
- Bend your neck forward slowly in a continuous downward motion toward your chest.
- Try to touch your chin to your chest or sternum.

THE OPTIMUM FLEXION ANGLE IS 40 DEGREES.

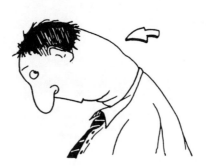

EXTENSION or LOOKING UP

From a central position, arch your neck upwards and look at the ceiling.

THE OPTIMUM EXTENSION ANGLE IS 70 DEGREES.

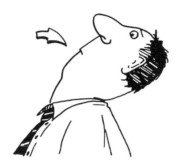

ROTATION or TURNING FROM SIDE TO SIDE

Patients generally experience greater mobility turning to one side or the other; i.e., from centre to right or from centre to left. Muscle tightness, overdevelopment of muscles, or injury will limit movement in one of the two directions. After practising the rotation exercises, compare the movement on both sides. Assess which side affords you greater comfort and flexibility.

THE OPTIMUM MOVEMENT WHEN ROTATING THE NECK TO ONE SIDE IS 90 DEGREES.

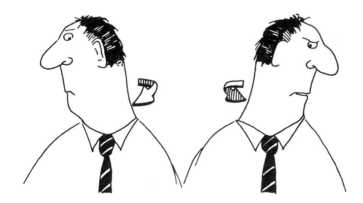

Movements that are frequently overlooked when exercising the neck are:

SIDE BENDING or LATERAL BENDING

- Stand still, without moving any portion of your upper or lower body.
- Keep the shoulders stable – do not move them.
- Bend your neck to the side and try to touch the lobe of your ear to one shoulder.
- Repeat on the opposite side and compare for flexibility – ability to achieve the goal of lobe-to-shoulder touching.

THE OPTIMUM MOVEMENT HERE SHOULD BE APPROXIMATELY 40 DEGREES.

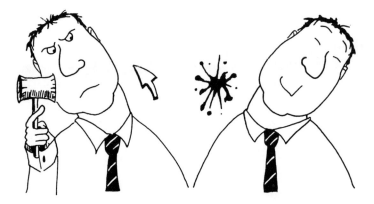

Now give yourself a critical appraisal. How well do you think you did? Did you experience any lack of mobility in your neck exercises?

If you experienced pain or restriction in the movement of your neck when performing these tests, it is important to **start a stretching program** immediately. If you could not turn your head to the right or to the left freely, practise the following:

- Slowly stretch the muscles of your neck by turning right (or left) as far as you can. Do not strain yourself – continue turning only to a point of restriction or pain.
- Hold this position for fifteen seconds, then slowly move your head back to the centre position.
- Repeat all of these exercises four times in the morning, afternoon and evening.

Remember, we want to stretch the neck, not to harm it. It is important not to strain forcefully beyond the point of restriction.

The same procedure can be used for restrictions in flexion/extension, or in lateral bending.

If you follow a daily regime of slowly stretching tightened muscles and ligaments, you will restore the normal movement of your neck.

4

Body Language: What is Pain?

*"Man is an apprentice. Pain is his master,
and no one understands who has not
suffered."*
ALFRED DE MARIGNY

The definition of pain according to the International Association for the Study of Pain is:

"Pain is an unpleasant sensory and emotional experience associated with actual or potential tissue damage or described in terms of such damage."

Pain is a message from the brain telling us that there is something wrong with the body.

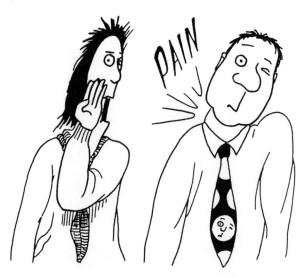

THAT'S NOT REAL PAIN.
IT'S JUST IN YOUR HEAD.

You can measure blood pressure or heart rate, and check the heart's function by use of an electrocardiogram (ECG), but a physiological measurement for pain does not exist.

However, what does exist are over **100** words used to describe pain, such as: gnawing, dull, sharp, stabbing, pulsing, gruelling, splitting, radiating, pounding, flickering, excruciating, searing and so forth. Research has shown that the more suffering people undergo, the more words they use to describe **pain**. As a result, the practitioner often measures pain by the words used to describe it. There is even a **McGill Pain Questionnaire (MPQ)** based on words, recognized internationally as a basic tool for assessing pain. While pain itself is not measurable, its physical effects in acute injury are. For example:

- increased pulse rate
- increased respiration rate
- increased blood pressure

Pain is also a source of negative stress. Stress has been shown to interfere with the healthy functioning of our **immune system**. The immune system is the body's front line defence in combatting illness and aiding the healing process.

In conclusion, although we cannot see or measure pain, it is **real**, not a figment of our imagination, and its effects are demonstrable.

5

Whiplash: A Modern-Day Curse

"What is done can't be undone."
SHAKESPEARE

It was the summer of 1967. I was travelling with my parents, older brother and sister on a day trip to the city of Nairobi approximately 300 miles away from our family home in Mombasa, East Africa.

The dawn was breaking over the lush jungles of the Serengeti National Park and so far the trip had been uneventful. Our Volkswagen was handling the bumpy roads of the Serengeti with ease. In the front seat of the car, mom and dad were talking quietly to one another, while the "kids" in the back were busy admiring the spectacular scenery – hoping to catch a glimpse of a lion or a cheetah on the horizon.

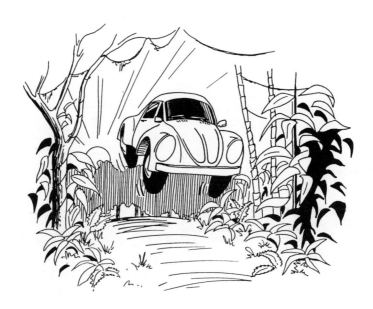

Suddenly, without warning, the tires blew out. Our car veered wildly out of control, became airborne and flipped over three times. The glass windows were ejected from their casings, yet strangely not one shattered! The car flipped and rolled for the third time, and came to rest on its side. My parents and all the children were turned into human projectiles as the force of the impact sent us hurtling through the twisted metal openings that only seconds before had secured the car's windows in place.

I remember a quiet hush descending over the scene of the accident. We slowly began picking ourselves up from the dusty road, each anxious to ensure the safety of the others. Miraculously, no one appeared to be injured. There were no signs of broken bones, scratches or blood on any of us. But, we were all holding our necks. Like a bad dream, or a surrealistic painting by Salvador Dali, the accident of seconds ago seemed unreal. But the pain in my neck was very **REAL!**

I did not know it then but I had sustained a Whiplash injury.

I was fortunate, however, as youth was on my side, and the warmth of the East African climate augured well in the healing process that would ensue. Yet even today I am plagued with the after-effects of the accident: physical and mental trauma, the regrettable "legacy" inherited by the victims of Whiplash, a legacy that no amount of compensation can ameliorate.

On the bright side of a negative injury, Whiplash is now a well-documented and accepted medical fact of life. Treatment modalities are by far superior to the "complete bed rest, epsom-salt baths, oil of wintergreen massages and drinking of large amounts of water" prescribed a mere 20 or 30 years ago.

Today, scientific, medical and engineering journals are featuring well-documented articles outlining the continuing research and findings about both physical and mental damages sustained in Whiplash injury, and about its treatment. Many articles point out that soft tissue injury of the neck and back is difficult to prove objectively. Pain is a very subjective or personal experience for the patient. Each of us has a different pain threshold, or tolerance to pain, making it difficult to generalize or quantify. Nonetheless, what has been established and what is being written about is the common thread in all Whiplash injuries – **the pain is real** and Whiplash victims experience pain in varying intensities.

As a direct result of the acceptance of Whiplash injury as a medical entity, many automobile manufacturers have responded positively. They have introduced into the marketplace technologically advanced automobiles featuring proper head restraints, lap/harness seatbelts and air bags. Many cars also feature the automatic onset of headlights as soon as the engine is started. The latter is particularly important, as many accidents occur during the day and when driving into the sun, for example, and the use of headlights can help to reduce the risk of accidents. Included in the growing list of measures provided by responsible manufacturers to prevent Whiplash are upgraded infant car seats for travelling "babes in arms."

As a result of these measures, injuries are often not as debilitating as they once were and practitioners are seeing a dramatic change for the better in the type and degree of Whiplash injuries.

Nevertheless, the diversity of symptoms, combined with the complexities of the patients' injuries and the subjective nature of pain, make **Whiplash a Modern-Day Curse!**

6

Whiplash – Its Symptoms: "The Many Faces of Eve" Syndrome

"We think in generalities, we live in detail."
ALFRED NORTH WHITEHEAD

Sixty to 70 percent of all Whiplash injuries result from a rear-end collision between two or more vehicles. The lead, or primary vehicle slows or stops in traffic, and is hit from behind by a second vehicle. The force of the impact will vary from accident to accident, depending on speed, styles of cars involved, etc. In the case of multi-vehicular pile-ups, the first and second vehicles set off a chain reaction and, in extreme cases, as many as 20 or more vehicles have been involved.

Other Whiplash injuries can occur as a result of "right angle" and "side-swipe" collisions.

The force of the colliding motor vehicles causes the neck to "whip" to and fro, damaging the neck's internal structures.

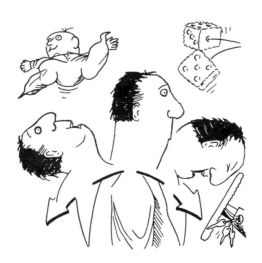

Different types of collisions cause specific types of injuries to various soft tissues; these are known as **soft tissue injuries**. Harm to the neck tissues may result in damage to the muscles, ligaments, blood vessels, nerves, discs, skin, pharynx, larynx, glands, and other body tissues.

Most practitioners will inform the patient that he or she has sustained a **mild, moderate or severe cervical strain/sprain**, which simply means that muscles and ligaments have been slightly stretched or partially torn in the neck.

However, like Eve, Whiplash wears many faces. There are times when the numerous symptoms of Whiplash become so confusing to the practitioner that he or she misdiagnoses and relegates the symptoms to a completely unrelated cause.

Many patients experience most of the symptoms. Others experience only some, but this does not necessarily invalidate the seriousness of the injuries.

Typical symptoms are:

- headaches
- neck/upper back pain
- nausea
- dizziness
- jaw pain
- ringing in the ears
- blurry vision
- insomnia
- imbalance
- tingling and numbness in fingers/arm
- fatigue
- depression
- hot/cold chills
- spasm
- stiffness
- difficulty swallowing
- weight fluctuations
- palpitations
- low back pain

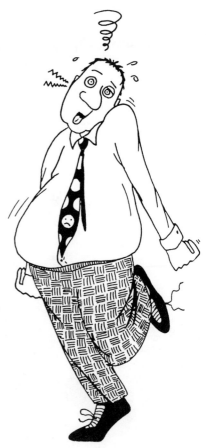

While generalizations about Whiplash injuries can be drawn from large population studies, Whiplash is still unique to the individual and requires consistent and standardized evaluating procedures.

For example, at hospital "A," the patient may be assured that everything is fine and told to go home and rest. Hospital "B" may have placed the patient in a neck collar or brace, prescribed medication/pain killers, and referred him or her for physiotherapy, therapeutic massage and a consultation with a specialist.

It is easy, therefore, to understand why inconsistency and lack of standardized evaluating procedures within many health disciplines can easily result in too little, too much or the wrong kind of treatment.

7

Whiplash: Factors Influencing its Extent and Severity

"We are confronted by a condition, not a theory."
GROVER CLEVELAND

1) **AGE OF PATIENT**
   Older patients are less flexible. Their tissues are not as elastic or resilient and cannot, therefore, withstand the force that travels through the neck at the moment of impact.

2) **SEX**
   Women seem to be more vulnerable to injury than men due to less muscular strength and supportive mass in the neck region.

3) **THE HEAD POSITION AT IMPACT** discussed in **Whiplash: Were Your Head and Neck Rotated?** (chapter 10, below).

4) **ANTICIPATION**
   Bracing oneself when anticipating an accident decreases the extent of soft tissue injury. Relaxed patients seem to be injured more severely in the neck region because, much like with a rag doll, the neck will "flop" around beyond the normal range of motion.

5) **PREVIOUS INJURIES, SURGERIES or OSTEOARTHRITIS**
   We will discuss these injuries in **The Osteoarthritic or Degenerative Neck** (chapter 15, below). However, there is no doubt that these conditions predispose an area to greater injury as compared to previously non-injured areas, or ones not subjected to previous surgery or degenerative osteoarthritic changes.

6)   TYPES OF VEHICLES COLLIDING
Smaller vehicles when struck by larger vehicles absorb a greater force on impact, and transmit this force through the occupant's neck.

7)   THE USE OF CAR RESTRAINTS
Improper use or non-use of harness/lap seatbelts and head restraints may increase injuries.

8)   THE ANGLE AND SPEED OF IMPACT
Although faster movement (as in a fast-impact accident) usually causes greater damage to the vehicle, it does not necessarily cause greater soft tissue injury in the Whiplash patient.

9)   THE POSITION AND SUPPORT OF THE SEAT-BACK
The angle or spring in the back of the car's seats will determine the amount of force travelling through the spine.

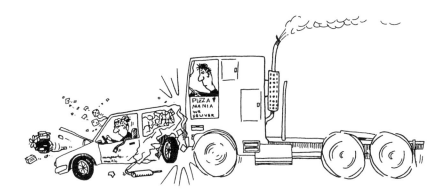

8

Your Whiplash Claim: Insurance, Adjusters and You

"One has information only to the extent to which one has tended to communicate one's experience."
H.S. SULLIVAN

In this book there are many references to neck injuries resulting from motor vehicle accidents. Current statistics indicate that approximately 75 percent of Whiplash injuries to the neck are the result of motor vehicle accidents. Therefore it is germane to the subject of neck pain treatment to examine the relationship between this treatment and the involvement of the insurance adjuster in the process.

In practise, an insurance adjuster can have some impact on the degree and method of treatment that an injured person may receive. Therefore it is important for the person who has been injured in a motor vehicle accident to understand the role of the insurance adjuster before beginning the claim-adjusting process.

The role of the insurance adjuster is an extremely important one. The adjuster is often the first person the patient will contact after the accident.

It is the adjuster's role to form a profile of the present nature of the patient's injuries, the extent of these injuries and their impact on the patient's occupation and lifestyle. Also, the long-term physical and mental ramifications will be taken into account.

Adjusters use a set of criteria to assist them in assessing injuries and establishing financial settlements.

SOME OF THE INFORMATION THE ADJUSTER RELIES UPON:

- The patient's personal statement (taken during the initial meeting with the adjuster) outlining his or her recollection of the sequence

of events just prior to, during and after the accident, and the symptoms experienced.
- The patient's occupation.
- Lifestyle endeavours of the patient (how active and in what areas).
- Assessment of damage sustained to the patient's car and other cars that may have been involved (the pattern of potential Whiplash injuries can often be evaluated by determining the area and extent of damage to the cars involved).
- Reports from the patient's health care practitioners and specialists to verify the amount of physical damage and the prognosis as to future disabilities.
- Statements from other parties involved and from witnesses to the accident.

The evaluation of the adjuster is of paramount importance to the patient's settlement. Apart from the payment for immediate treatment for the Whiplash injury to the neck, consideration is given for the treatment of potential future recurrence of symptoms related to the injury.

The claimant may or may not accept the offer from the insurance company. He or she may think that the injuries are more serious than assessed by the adjuster. This subjective thinking may result from discussions with well-intentioned friends, other compensated claimants and "facts" read from newspapers.

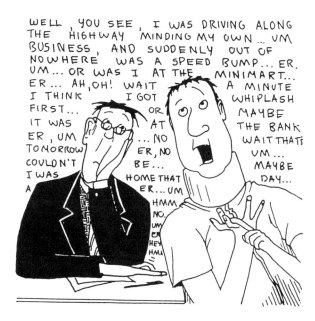

At this point, the case may go to litigation and lawyers representing both the claimant and the insurance company will compile a detailed profile of the accident and the injuries sustained.

Depending on the severity of the neck injuries and the overall complexities of the case, this process may continue over many months or even years before a settlement is reached.

The onerous nature of the claims process itself has often been described by patients suffering from Whiplash-related neck injury as a **"pain in the neck!"**

9

The When and Where of
Whiplash Occurrence

*"Events do not come, they are there and we
encounter them on our way."*
ARTHUR S. EDDINGTON

Accidents causing Whiplash **usually** take place:
- in suburban areas
- at relatively low speeds
- during daylight hours
- at intersections

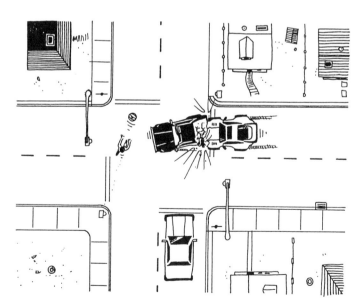

10

Whiplash: Were Your Head and Neck Rotated?

"A problem well stated is a problem half solved."
CHARLES F. KETTERING

Following a Whiplash injury, the majority of patients will complain of one-sided pain; e.g., a left or right-sided headache and right arm or left shoulder discomfort. Rarely will a practitioner observe a complete **bilateral symptomatology** (equal pain on both sides).

Biomechanically, a rotational injury connected with Whiplash is more serious compared to what is called the "straight-positioned" Whiplash. A "normal" neck will extend or move backward up to 70 degrees.

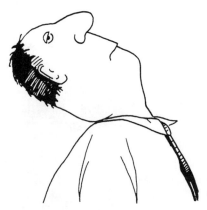

NORMAL EXTENSION

If the neck is rotated 45 degrees to either side and extended backward, the range of healthy extension decreases by 50 percent to a mere 35 degrees.

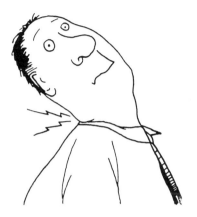

HYPEREXTENSION ROTATION

As illustrated above, the decrease of neck extension along with rotation increases the degree of soft tissue damage by pushing on the joints at the back of the neck. This type of hyperextension causes damage to the soft tissues, blood vessels and spinal canal.

Rotational Whiplash injuries to the upper neck can easily damage the **vertebral artery**, which travels through the neck vertebrae supplying blood to the brain tissues. With this type of injury there may be compression of the vertebral artery, and much like the twisting of a garden hose which cuts off the flow of water, the supply of blood to the brain is decreased. The result is a lack of oxygen to the brain and a one-sided headache.

One-sided head and neck symptoms should alert your practitioner to rule out rotational hyperextension injury as the cause of the problem.

Questioning by the insurance adjuster or the practitioner after the accident will often reveal that the patient's head, neck and/or torso were rotated at the time of the accident. It is not unusual to hear a patient state:

- "I saw the car coming in my rear-view mirror."
- "I was looking down adjusting the dial on the radio."
- "I was looking at the sidewalk waiting for pedestrians to cross the road."

These statements indicate a variety of positions which place the head and neck in a rotated stance at the time of impact.

TREATMENT AND PREVENTION:

In the acute phase, **never** turn or rotate your neck suddenly in the same direction it was in during the accident.

When experiencing head and neck pain as a result of rotational neck injury, in the acute phase **avoid** any exercise in which you turn and extend your neck backward. This will cause further "pinching" of the damaged artery. Instead, exercise by turning the neck in the opposite direction, by flexing or turning the head and neck tissues forward.

Usually, the headache is on the same side as the injury. The following exercise will open up pinched tissues, and allow an increase in blood flow to the brain.

- Forward bend or flex and then slowly rotate the head and neck to the opposite side of the head pain.
- Hold this contraction for 15 seconds.
- Come back to the centre slowly, and repeat four times.

Do this exercise morning, afternoon and evening.

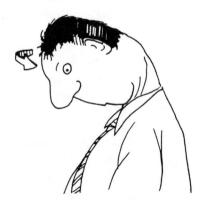

11

Whiplash – Head Restraints: Are Yours Adjusted Correctly?

"He that will not apply new remedies must expect new evils, for time is the greatest innovator."
FRANCIS BACON

Seatbelts (harness and lap types), adjustable head restraints and air bags are becoming standard features in most vehicles.

Statistics show that the correct use of seatbelts and air bags has significantly decreased the fatality rate.

Front-seat head restraints are compulsory in all cars and are now featured in rear seats of some vehicles. Head restraints were originally called headrests and, as the name implied, most people considered them to be a luxury feature rather than a safety item. When adjusted correctly, the head restraint will protect the neck from severe damage experienced in a hyperextensive Whiplash injury.

To gain maximum protection from the use of head restraints, the top of the head restraint should be level with the top of the ears. In the event of an accident, this will protect the base of the skull and neck, preventing the hyperextensive motion of the neck.

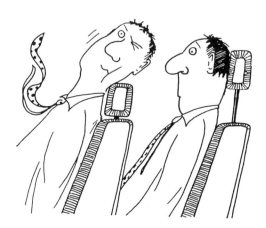

The neck, when in a hyperextensive movement, can travel well beyond the 70-degree normal extension or backward movement, thus causing the tearing of **soft tissues**. Head restraints will limit the motion of the neck to considerably below the 70-degree range, preventing severe damage in many Whiplash cases.

12

"Oh, My Splitting Headache!"

"Any ache but heartache, any pain but in the head."

Many of you who have chosen to read this book will immediately flip to the **"headache"** section. Why is this? The reason, unlike the diagnosis, is quite simple. Countless thousands of you have suffered the miseries of this "Hallowe'en Syndrome." And, much like a Hallowe'en reveller, headaches come in many disguises....

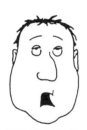

TENSION HEADACHE

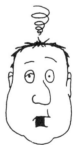

POST-TRAUMATIC HEADACHE

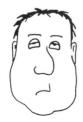

LOW BLOOD SUGAR HEADACHE

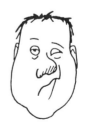

ALLERGY HEADACHE

This complicates the picture, making categorical diagnosis difficult to pin-point. So let us explore some common causes of headaches, and several factors influencing the severity of symptoms.

Tension headaches and post-traumatic headaches are two of the most prevalent headache disorders. But this does not make them any less severe or painful than headaches from other origins. Tension and post-traumatic headaches are the direct result of bio-mechanical and physiological changes in the neck region. In lay person's language, "bio-mechanical" and "physiological" simply mean changes in the joint movements and normal functions of the body.

With tension headaches, the patient experiences a generalized ache at the base of the skull or head, originating from the neck, called cephalgia. Often there is an accompanying tightness in the upper back muscles. A hot bath, the comforting warmth of a shower, or an aspirin, sometimes in combination, may diminish the pain or relieve the headache before it takes hold. Often simply resting the neck on a contoured pillow will alleviate symptoms. However, when a person is undergoing psychological stress, such as from an argument with a spouse or children demanding attention, the pain in the neck will increase proportionately to the level of tension. Like ripples from a pebble thrown into a pond, the headache worsens as one set of circumstances builds on the other, resulting in spasms of the neck muscles, tissues tightening and the full-blown headache syndrome descending on the hapless victim. But there is hope. Relief is on the way!

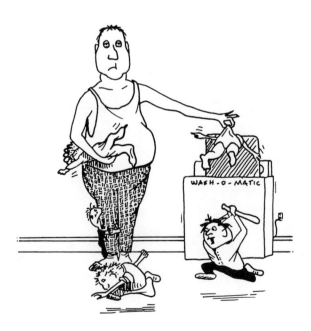

Post-traumatic headaches are often related to motor vehicle accidents or Whiplash injury.

In a typical case there is **absolutely no history** of previous headache. Pain is located primarily on one side of the neck and head, and may radiate into the patient's eye, ear, jaw or temple. In relation to the injuries, movement of the neck in certain directions may increase or conversely decrease the pain. At times the pain is so severe that nausea may result and the patient's vision may be temporarily affected. Like the tide, the pain may ebb and flow, sweeping over the patient and causing varying degrees of discomfort. As in the case of tension headaches, stress can aggravate a post-traumatic headache. The pain is hard to endure, and aggressive in nature, moving quickly to full-blown symptoms of migraine.

This type of condition is usually the result of an injury to the top portion of the neck with damage to the upper nerves which exit from the spinal cord. In many cases, there is a compression of the vertebral artery at the base of the skull (which is a crucial blood-supply artery to the brain) and pain ensues. Insufficient blood supply to one side of the head results in bizarre one-sided head and neck symptoms such as: dizziness, blurry vision, ringing in the ears, feeling off-balance and one-sided headaches at the temple.

TREATMENT AND PREVENTION:

The following exercises will assist in decreasing the stiffness and tension developed in the upper back and neck muscles that causes headaches.

EXERCISE 1

- Sit or stand tall and gently extend your neck backward in a smooth arc.
- Hold the stretch for 5 seconds and repeat 10 times.

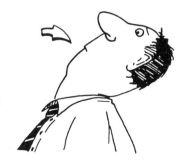

EXERCISE 2

- Stand tall with your arms beside you.
- Slowly rotate your shoulders forward in a circular motion, then gently make larger circles. Repeat this 10 times.
- Now reverse the direction of motion and repeat 10 times.

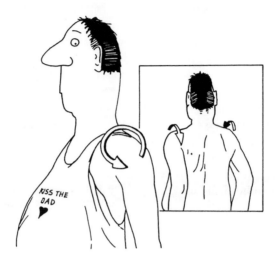

EXERCISE 3

- Stand tall and retract your chin backward into the neck.
- Interlock your hands behind the head, and by applying even pressure, gently push your head into the palms of your hands.
- Hold this contraction for 5 seconds, with no movement. Repeat this exercise 10 times.

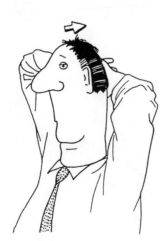

EXERCISE 4

- Stand tall with your arms beside you.
- Slowly shrug both your shoulders up toward your ears.
- Hold this for 5 seconds and repeat 10 times.

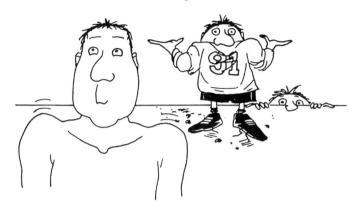

Complete this exercise program by resting on the floor with a rolled-up towel supporting the neck for 5 minutes. Do all these exercises a minimum of twice daily until there is relief.

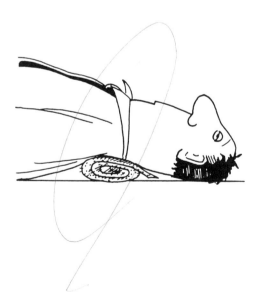

13

Whiplash – Neck Collars:
Do They Help?

*"Progress is a nice word. But change is its
motivator and change has its enemies."*
ROBERT F. KENNEDY

Almost every patient involved in a car accident who has sustained a "serious" Whiplash injury is taken to the emergency room of a hospital, and fitted with a neck collar or brace. These collars range from extra-soft to extra-firm support structures.

Theoretically, the collar acts as a splint to avoid movement of the muscles and joints of the neck, in order to limit aggravation of the damaged area and to provide neck support. However, in practise, the collar allows the neck considerable mobility. Collars can be cumbersome, painful and difficult to tighten without a "choking" sensation. Using the most commonly prescribed cervical collars, it is not possible to splint the more than 37 movable joints of the neck. As a result of the stress on the neck from the collar, the pressure on inflamed neck muscles intensifies the pain and aggravates symptoms. In nearly all cases, rather than helping to ease the pain, the collars are described by patients as being "agony to wear."

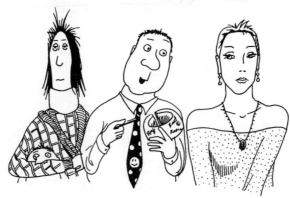

WILL YOU SIGN MY COLLAR?

Injured patients with a cervical collar will often drive a vehicle. Unless it is absolutely necessary, this is not recommended. The vulnerabilities of the injuries, combined with the wearing of a collar or brace, will inevitably present problems to the drivers, particularly, when they attempt to position their neck in order to look over their shoulder to see beyond the car's "blind spot." Drivers with cervical collars are a hazard not only to themselves but to other innocent drivers and passengers.

Professionally, I am against the use of cervical collars because they do, in fact, exacerbate muscle and joint stiffness and are counter-productive to the healing process they are supposed to promote. Furthermore, the most up-to-date scientific research has revealed that movement and exercise of the neck in the earliest stages following the trauma results in the fastest and most effective recovery. Weeks of bed-rest and the use of neck collars will weaken the neck's support muscles, decrease mobility and prolong symptoms of the disorder.

If the patient's symptoms are severe and the neck cannot withstand the pressure of sitting or standing, then the head and neck should rest on a pillow. I would recommend a collar as a cervical "crutch" only in extreme circumstances – for example: a patient being removed from the scene of an accident, an injured bride or groom who isn't willing to delay a wedding, a student who cannot be excused from final exams, or an employee whose services are truly indispensable.

TREATMENT AND PREVENTION:

Instead of the collar, I recommend the following:
- Lie on your back with a rolled-up towel, the size of a fist, supporting the neck.
- Gently withdraw the chin into the neck (to the point of discomfort).
- Hold this contraction for 5 seconds and repeat 10 times, five times daily until the acute pain subsides.

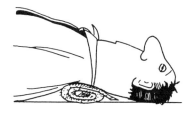 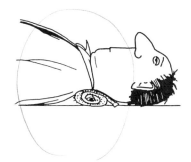

As your condition improves, slowly incorporate the exercises outlined in **How Well Does Your Neck Move?** (chapter 3), performing them while lying down.

14

X-Rays: Radiographic Examination

"A disease known is half cured."
THOMAS FULLER

X-rays are important in diagnosing trauma to the neck region. The majority of patients sustaining a Whiplash injury will require a complete x-ray profile of their neck. Similarly, patients experiencing chronic or ongoing neck pain, headaches or referred pain should have x-rays taken if their symptoms persist. X-rays will assist practitioners in detecting underlying pathology.

WHAT DOES A NECK X-RAY REVEAL?

In Whiplash cases, up to seven different x-rays of the neck may be taken, while for other problems a practitioner will requisition a minimum of two views in total (the front and side of the patient's neck).

A normal neck x-ray will show seven vertebrae, separated by disc spaces that are even, with uniformly aligned joints and an **optimum lordotic** forward curve.

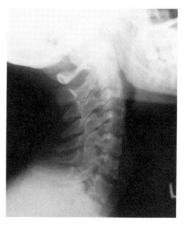

X-ray of an **OPTIMUM LORDOTIC** neck curve.

Patients who have sustained a Whiplash injury will show damage to neck ligaments, and a straightening of the neck curve or a **loss** or **reversal of lordosis**. A **straight neck curve** may appear directly after the accident or over a period of time. It is not always painful, but may eventually lead to osteoarthritic or degenerative changes in the neck.

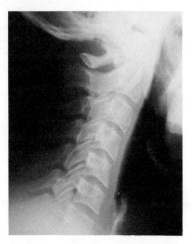

X-ray of an **ABNORMAL STRAIGHTENING** of the neck.

Neck x-rays **will not** show any direct damage to the muscles, nor will they show the discs between the vertebrae. However, they **will** reveal the narrowing of the disc spaces between vertebrae, and osteoarthritic changes. Depending on the x-ray evaluation and any other problems detected, further and more sophisticated diagnostic testing may be required, such as:

COMPUTERIZED AXIAL TOMOGRAPHY (CAT SCAN):

A non-invasive procedure employing the use of a computer, which is so precise it can take pictures of cross-sections of the spine no more than one-fifth of an inch in thickness.

MYELOGRAM:

This procedure is used to verify possible protrusions into the spinal canal, such as disc prolapses, tumors, and arthritic lesions. A dye is injected into the space surrounding the spinal cord and x-rays are taken. If the dye does not flow through, or is blocked, this indicates damage to the area.

MAGNETIC RESONANCE IMAGING (MRI):

A relatively new non-invasive imaging technique that produces cross-sectional pictures of the head, body and spine without the use of x-rays or radioactive materials. The technique has no known side effects.

DISCOGRAM:

This involves the use of radio-opaque dye injected directly into the disc. If the x-ray shows dye leaking from the disc, this procedure then confirms the diagnosis of disc disease.

In summary, the x-ray, physical and postural examinations, and symptoms outlined by the patient will all assist the practitioner in designing a specific and individual course of treatment. Patients may also request a viewing of their x-rays, and an explanation of any changes detected and how these changes may affect them now and in the future.

15

The Osteoarthritic or Degenerative Neck

"Wounds heal and become scars. But scars grow with us."
STANISLAW LEC

For many people the term **ARTHRITIS** conjures up a vision of crippled, swollen fingers, excruciating pain and the total disability often inherited by sufferers of **rheumatoid arthritis**.

The chances are excellent that you do **not** have this type of arthritis in your neck.

There are a hundred varieties of arthritis and, like viruses, they affect different parts of the body, causing symptoms unique to the specific strain experienced by the patient.

The most common arthritic neck condition is the **osteoarthritic** or **degenerative neck syndrome**. In this instance there is a disintegration of the joint and disc surfaces caused by trauma to the region, overuse, misuse or

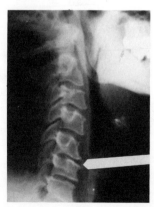

White arrow indicates area of **OSTEOARTHRITIC CHANGES**

faulty posture. The spaces between the vertebrae wear and tear, setting up a fertile environment for the onset of the osteoarthritic neck. But this does not mean in all cases that the patient will be plagued by a lifetime of pain and discomfort. Further, contrary to popular belief, it is a known medical fact that osteoarthritis does not always cause pain.

This disorder does not occur overnight; blood tests will not confirm its presence; and verification depends on the use of x-rays.

Often x-rays – in the absence of symptoms – are not taken and, even when they are, it is difficult to confirm when the arthritic changes began.

Unfortunately, patients with no previous symptoms who have this condition, and who are involved in a motor vehicle accident, may find that the accident triggers a physical chain reaction of painful flare-ups and osteoarthritic distress. In essence, the trauma of the accident has awakened the disorder from its period of dormancy.

It is not unusual for the osteoarthritic patient to experience painful flare-ups in damp, cold or rainy weather. This phenomenon is caused by changes in the barometric pressure, which causes a "compressive effect" on the internal joints. The joints resist the compressive effect in an attempt to achieve equilibrium, and this causes pain.

Arthritic changes of the neck usually indicate abnormal bio-mechanical joint movement, with tenderness of the surrounding tissues. It is extremely important to adjust the bio-mechanics of the neck to prevent further wear, tear and degradation of the neck tissues.

A unique finding in our practise has been that patients with skin-fold markings on the back of their necks that are tender, with restricted joint movement when palpated, will consistently show osteoarthritic changes on x-ray examination.

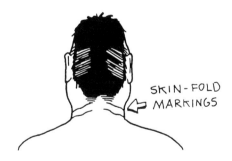

SKIN-FOLD MARKINGS

TREATMENT AND PREVENTION:

People with osteoarthritis of the neck must exercise with care. They may practise the following exercises but they must do them **more fre-**

quently with an emphasis on a **gentle approach** complemented by an understanding of their **osteoarthritic** condition.

Gentle rotation and side-bending neck exercises will increase the mobility of the stiffened joints.

EXERCISE 1

- Stand or sit tall and slowly rotate your neck to the left as far as it will go without causing pain.
- Hold for 15 seconds, then do this in the opposite direction.
- Repeat this exercise 10 times, twice daily.

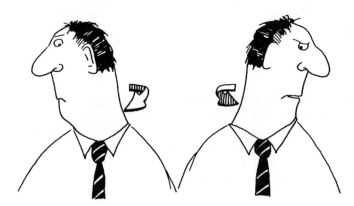

EXERCISE 2

- Stand tall and gently stretch your neck sideways in an attempt to touch your shoulder.
- Hold for 15 seconds and stretch in the opposite direction.
- Do this exercise 10 times, twice daily.

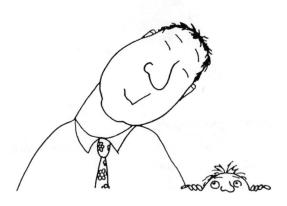

EXERCISE 3

  - Stand tall and interlock your hands in front of your forehead.
  - Apply equal pressure forward with the head and backward with the hands and hold the contraction for 5 seconds.
  - Repeat this exercise 10 times, twice daily.

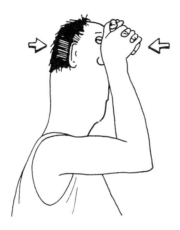

EXERCISE 4

  - Sitting or standing, interlock your hands over your head, and apply equal pressure upward and downward, and do not move.
  - Hold the contraction for 5 seconds. Repeat 10 times, twice daily.

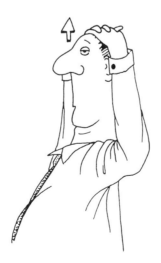

16

Trigger Points: What Are They and How Do They Influence Pain?

"If they say it's there, question them; if you feel it's there, believe them."
S.S. NEEL

Trigger points, myofascial pain syndrome, and fibrositis are long names used to identify a small pea-like structure in the muscle or ligamentous tissue.

This tiny ball can radiate excruciating pain to other parts of the body. Perhaps a good percentage of the readers have experienced pain from this trigger point: your practitioner is palpating or massaging the soft tissues of your neck and back when suddenly, as the hand is rubbed over a muscle, it hits this pea-like mass. The pain is hot and electric, you jump and cry out, or at least want to!

The cause of myofascial pain syndrome is a repeated insult and trauma to certain muscle fibres, causing them to become ropy in texture. This results in a decrease of blood and oxygen being delivered to the tissues, instigating pain and discomfort. The spin-off effect is that the body develops a so-called "negative cycle"; the pain causes the muscles to tighten even further, creating more pain – a vicious circle of agony.

During times of physical and psychological stress, trigger points can and do flare-up. They may not cause pain at the point of origin, but may direct or refer the pain to other regions of the body. For example, a trigger point in the upper trapezius muscle, located at the upper mid-back, will activate pain in the base of the skull, head, or eye.

Trigger points are extremely annoying to the practitioner, because they cannot be "objectively" diagnosed by means of x-ray or ultrasound. Fortunately, the practitioner can detect them by touch and treat them, and they are not permanent.

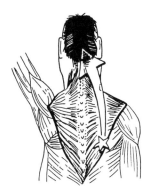

A trigger point in the upper trapezius muscle referring pain.

TREATMENT AND PREVENTION:

To alleviate the stress or pain associated with **myofascial pain syndrome**, perform the following exercises and seek treatment from a trained practitioner.

EXERCISE 1

- Stand tall and draw your chin backward into your neck.
- Simultaneously, draw your shoulder blades together and lift your head up as if an imaginary balloon is pulling your head up toward the ceiling.
- Hold this contraction for 5 seconds and repeat 10 times.

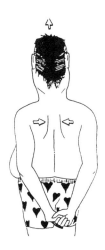

EXERCISE 2

- Interlock your hands behind your head.
- Retract or draw your chin **into** your neck. **Do not pull the chin down**.
- With your chin drawn in, push your arms backwards, bringing your shoulder blades as close together as possible.
- Hold this contraction for 5 seconds. Repeat it 10 times.

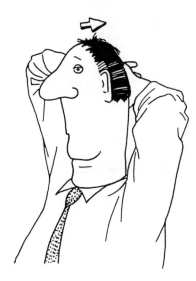

Perform these exercises morning, afternoon and evening to strengthen the muscles of the upper back and neck.

17

Radiculopathy: Nerve Root Damage and Referred Pain

"Where it is , is not where you think it is."
S.S. NEEL

There are **31** pairs of nerve roots in the spinal column – each pair sandwiched between two vertebrae, the latter being separated by the gelatinous mass known as a **disc**. Nerve roots exit horizontally from both sides of the vertebrae through small openings no more than a centimetre wide, called the **intervertebral foramen** or the **IVF**. It is at this juncture that the **nerve roots** become known as the **spinal nerves**. Working together synergistically, spinal nerves provide sensation and power to the muscles and skin.

Damage to a disc may precipitate a narrowing of the **IVF** space, causing significant pressure and irritation on the spinal nerve root as it exits between the vertebrae. However, it is not at this source that pain will be experienced by the patient. The pain will be referred by a nerve from the damaged area to the specific location where the spinal nerves innervate or provide sensation and power to the tissues.

As illustrated below, each nerve root originating from the neck (numbered C5 to C8) has the ability to affect a different part of the arm, forearm and hand. In some cases the nerve root irritation may cause numbness, pain, tingling, muscle weakness or a combination of these symptoms.

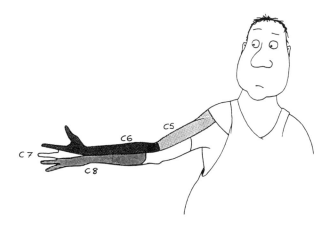

Patients who have a pre-existing **osteoarthritic disc degenerative disease** of the neck and who later suffer a Whiplash injury may experience further narrowing of the **IVF**. This is important because only a minor disruption to the disc is necessary to cause significant pressure and irritation to the spinal nerve root. Therefore, any disruptive condition must be of concern and warrants a thorough follow-up by the practitioner.

Only when a narrowed **IVF** has been confirmed by x-ray, and there are symptoms of referred pain, can the diagnosis of **radiculopathy** be made.

After diagnosis, treatment should be pursued immediately because continued pressure on the **nerve root** will produce loss of function of that particular nerve, as well as muscle weakness and diminished sensation. In the worst-case scenario, if several nerve roots are involved, a patient may be unable to perform a simple task such as lifting a glass to his or her mouth.

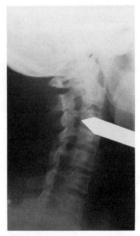

White arrow indicates narrowing of **IVF**.

TREATMENT AND PREVENTION:

Pain radiating in one arm, hand or finger can indicate damage or narrowing of the **IVF** on that side of the body.

- Side-bend your neck to the opposite and pain-free shoulder. This will increase or expand the **IVF** opening and decrease the pressure on the "pinched" or pinching nerve.
- For example, if the pain is in the left arm, side-bend your neck slowly to the right shoulder to your maximum stretching ability, or to the onset of pain or discomfort. This will increase or expand the **IVF** opening, and decrease the pressure on the **spinal nerve root**.
- Hold this stretch for 15 seconds and repeat 4 times.

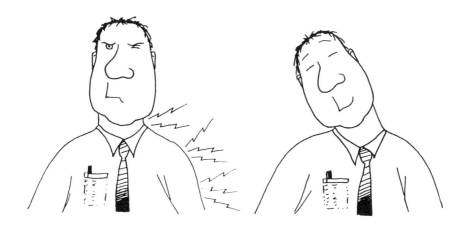

Practise this exercise in the morning, afternoon and evening.

Referred pain in the arm or shoulder does not always result from damage to the **IVF**. In certain cases pain can originate from a dysfunction of the heart, gall bladder or soft tissues. Unless you have a positive diagnosis by a trained practitioner that you are experiencing symptoms of damage to the **intervertebral foramen (IVF)**, do not undertake the above exercise. A diagnosis by your practitioner is both warranted and recommended.

18

Hypermobility: Are You A Grinder?

"Too little movement is bad. Too much movement is worse."
S.S. NEEL

Are you the neck-crunching equivalent of a knuckle cracker? In other words do you turn your neck in quick, jerky movements, making it "**pop**," to release a feeling of stiffness?

Does your neck feel better momentarily, but within minutes more painful and rigid? If so, you have just taken another self-defeating "**crack**" at trying to ease the pain and tension of an already traumatized neck. **Don't do it!** And, while some people hear a cracking or popping sound when they turn their necks in a normal manner, the noisy grinding sounds experienced by both the "**flicker**" and the regular neck turner are indications of an abnormal hypermobile neck.

Why does the neck become hypermobile? Let's look to the circus for an example. Most of us have watched in awe as a fearless lion tamer enters a barred cage in the centre of a sawdust ring. A door to a tunnel-like structure pulls open and several snarling lions bound out. Often they are reluctant to take their places on the oversized stools in the cage. We note that the lion tamer is brandishing a long, slim, leather bullwhip, making exaggerated circles over his head. Suddenly, with lightning speed, he brings the handle of the whip parallel to his shoulder. And, in the same fluid motion, he extends his wrist slightly backwards propelling the tongue of the whip to the ground. The force of the whip cutting through the air makes a familiar "**whooshing**" sound. In the split second before the whip contacts terra firma, the lion tamer exerts another hearty wrist flick.

We hear a loud "**crack**," and in a microsecond he reverses the forward thrust to a backward motion, returning the whip to his shoulder level. He may repeat this forward/backward motion in grandiose fashion several

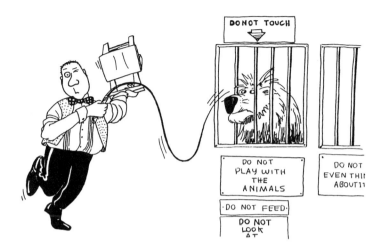

times – slight wrist extension backward, forward flick, whoosh, crack, wrist flick, backward thrust, wrist flick, forward thrust, whoosh, crack, etc.

Imagine for a moment that you are in a car when your vehicle is rear-ended by another. At the moment of collision your neck parallels the whip as it torques to and fro beyond its normal limits, until the cycle of movement caused by the crash ceases. And, like the leather of the well-used bullwhip, the girdle-style support mechanism of the neck ligaments is stretched by the force, setting the stage for **hypermobility** of this region.

Initially, the body's natural protective mechanism will tighten the neck's soft tissues to protect them and to avoid further damage. The tightening results in pain and limited flexibility. At this point, when the acute pain has subsided, many patients will attempt to increase neck motion by repeatedly and rapidly turning their neck from side to side. They usually hear an audible "**pop**" and a sudden burst of what they perceive to be warmth and energy in the neck area. Due to the temporary feelings of relief, patients erroneously believe they have mastered a "**self-alignment**" of the neck. Nothing could be further from the truth. The "**popping**" sound is **not an alignment of the neck structure** but the release of nitrogenous gases between the vertebral joints and, on occasion, the snapping/cracking sound is the result of stretched ligaments that are noisily overlapping. What this measure has accomplished is a worsening of the condition.

Whereas controlled, directed movement of neck vertebral joints by a trained practitioner is therapeutic, excessive and random motion results in overly slack neck muscles and ligaments. Like a worn elastic band, these soft tissues, normally supportive and flexible, lose their natural **elasticity**: the tissues cease to coil or spring back efficiently and rapidly, head and neck posture is distorted, and optimum control is diminished – resulting in popping, cracking and grinding noises with the slightest movement of the neck.

TREATMENT AND PREVENTION:

The objective of the following **isometric exercises** (the act of tensing one set of muscles against another) is to strengthen the muscles and ligaments of the neck and to aid in restoring the integrity of the damaged tissues. But nothing can take the place of avoiding the self-defeating actions of "cracking," "flicking" or "popping" the neck.

EXERCISE 1

- Stand tall and interlock your hands over your head.
- Apply equal pressure upward with your head and downward with your hands.
- Hold contraction for 5 seconds. Repeat 10 times, twice daily.

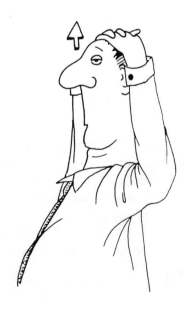

EXERCISE 2

- Stand tall and interlock your hands in front of your forehead.
- Applying equal pressure both forward with the head and backward with your hands, hold the contraction for 5 seconds.
- Repeat this exercise 10 times, twice daily.

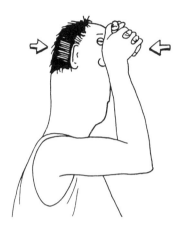

EXERCISE 3

- Bracing the side of the face with your palm, gently apply equal pressure into the palm with your face.
- Hold this contraction for 5 seconds. Repeat 10 times, twice daily.

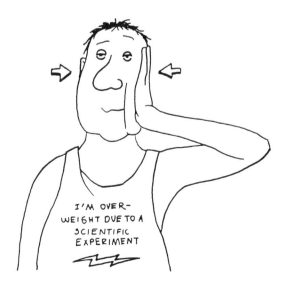

19

Prognosis: How Well Will I Be?

"You can never plan the future by the past."
EDMUND BURKE

We often hear health practitioners use the word "**prognosis**," as in "the prognosis is. . . ." But what does it mean?
According to the **Blakiston's GOULD Medical Dictionary**

PROGNOSIS (prog-no'-sis) *is a prediction as to the probable course and outcome of a disease, injury, or developmental abnormality in a patient, based on general knowledge of such conditions, as well as on specific information and exercise of clinical judgment in the particular case.*

Accurate diagnosis is of paramount importance; however, **prognosis** as to the probable course and outcome of a disease or injury is the cornerstone of effective long-term treatment. Incorrect prognosis can be a disaster for the patient, as the most effective methods available will not be used to assist in the patient's rehabilitation and recovery from injury or disease.

Recovery can best be defined as a return to a state of rest, equilibrium, or health from a state of fatigue, stress, or illness.

The patient's primary concerns are:
- How long will it take to get better?
- When will day-to-day activities be resumed in both leisure and work-related pursuits?

The answers to such concerns depend upon:
- The extent of physical and psychological damage caused by the injury or disorder.
- Treatment methods used.

While patients want a full recovery from their neck injury and pain, the reality is that only "**functional recovery**" is achieved in most cases.

Patients with **functional recovery** from a neck injury will become pain-free. They will return to work, but once their neck has been traumatized, the theory of the "weakest link in a chain" becomes their body's reality.

The injured neck, notwithstanding other medical problems, is weakened. Symptoms of distress will be aggravated by physical and emotional stressors, **incorrect exercise**, over-exertion of job-related functions (lifting, moving, heavy machinery operation, or sitting hunched-up in front of a word processor), for example. Even weather conditions such as rain, dampness, cold and snow have the potential to exacerbate or exaggerate symptoms, building to a flare-up of distress at the original site of injury. It is not unusual for the same area to be injured repeatedly, because like the parallel weak link in a chain, although healed, the tissues can never be "mended" or restructured to their original strength. Frequent injury will also determine the severity of neck pain and its recurrence.

To alleviate physical stress to weakened or damaged soft neck tissues, follow the exercises in the specific chapters related to your type of injury. They will assist you in maximizing your recovery potential.

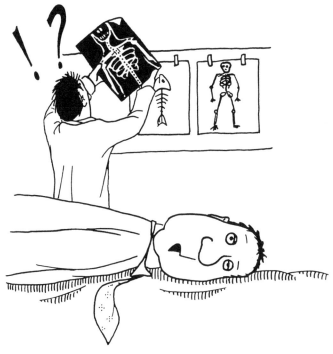

AM I EVER GOING TO GET BETTER, DOC?

20

Pillow Talk: Choosing A Neck Pillow

"Don't put a healthy head on a sick pillow."

B y the time most of us reach the age of 60 our neck and head will have been supported by a pillow for over 20 years. That is equal to approximately 240 months; 7,300 days; 175,200 hours; 10,512,000 minutes and 630,720,000 or **SIX HUNDRED AND THIRTY MILLION, SEVEN HUNDRED AND TWENTY THOUSAND SECONDS.**

When perceived in this light it is rather amazing how little thought or time we spend in choosing the right pillow. A pillow is **NOT** just a pillow. It is a structure that should offer optimum support to the tissues of the neck to ensure comfort, high quality sleeping patterns (prolonged disturbed sleep or lack of sleep can cause psychiatric disturbances), as well as a healthy neck!

Despite the importance to the human condition of finding the right pillow, there is little scientific literature available on the subject and none in the department stores. Most of us are forced to choose our favourite pillow by trial and error.

However, there are plenty of pillow types, such as:
- the soft/hard pillow
- the contour pillow
- the bean-filled pillow
- the air-filled pillow
- the rolled-up towel
- the cervical pillow
- the wedge pillow
- the feather pillow
- the futon pillow
- the goose-down pillow
- the foam pillow
- the loose foam-chip pillow
- the 100%-cotton stuffed hypoallergenic pillow

As well, many people will use the crook of their arm as a headrest ir of a pillow, causing neck, upper arm and shoulder pain. And from our society's perspective perhaps the most unusual "pillows" would be the indented stones used by a number of tribes in Africa.

When selecting the perfect pillow there are four important factors to keep in mind:

1. height
2. comfort
3. support structure
4. conformity to the neck structure

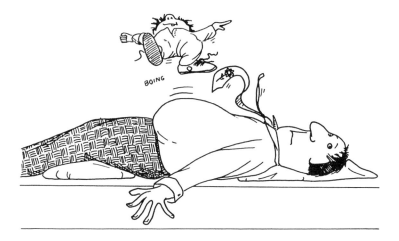

All factors considered, the pillow must be one that suits your individual needs. It is rare to find two people who, even with identical neck structures, would agree on the same type of pillow. What we do know is that people who have problems with their neck through bio-mechanical, postural changes or trauma should be x-rayed, so that the right kind of support can be prescribed by the practitioner.

TREATMENT AND PREVENTION:

Some people like to stagger two pillows to support the upper back and neck to a slightly flexed position while they read in bed or watch television. If they already have a slouched or hunched forward posture, this will only exaggerate the out-of-line position of the neck and back. People who have lost the lordotic curve in the neck and have a straight neck often complain of neck pain following a night's sleep.

Do this exercise daily before sleeping, to reinforce, mobilize and help restore the normal lordotic curve of the neck and remove the pain:
- Lie on your back with a towel rolled up to the size of your fist placed under your neck.
- Retract or draw your chin backward (making a double chin), pushing your neck into the towel.
- Hold for 10 seconds. Repeat 10 times.

You may sleep all night with the towel under your neck, but a proper pillow is recommended.

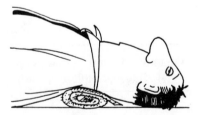 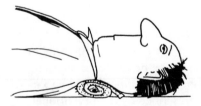

21

Should You Apply Cold or Heat?

"Cold is inimical to the bones, the teeth, the nerves, the brain and the spinal marrow, but heat is beneficial."
HIPPOCRATES

Many patients attending our clinic have utilized either cold or heat therapy to reduce their neck pain or spasm.

Every health practitioner has a favourite "treatment of choice." There is always a time when one treatment is more effective than another. Here are your options:

COLD

What does cold do to the body tissues?
1. Decreases the blood flow to the tissues initially
2. Reduces pain and tension in muscle tissues
3. Decreases swelling and inflammation
4. Has an anaesthetic and analgesic effect
5. Reduces the messages sent by nerves

HEAT

What does heat do to the body tissues?
1. Increases blood flow to the tissues
2. Reduces dull or chronic pain
3. Has an analgesic effect
4. Increases fluids and swelling in tissues

SEQUENTIAL THERAPY

The following outlines therapies which are utilized sequentially following neck injury, whether the trauma is minor or major.

Phase I – COLD

Apply cold to all new traumatic or acute injuries. Cold is applied for a maximum of 10-15 minutes every two hours. This decreases pain, swelling and inflammation. Continue this treatment for 24 to 48 hours or until the sharp pain and swelling decreases.

Phase II – COLD/HEAT

Alternating cold/heat application creates a pumping affect within tissues. Twenty-five minutes of alternating cold/hot therapy consisting of 5 minutes cold, 5 minutes hot; 5 minutes cold, 5 minutes hot; 5 minutes cold, is effective in decreasing tissue swelling, as this process removes the build-up of waste products in the damaged tissues.

Phase III – HEAT

The soothing warmth of heat is preferred by most patients to treat their neck injury. **It is also the most overused and misused therapy. HEAT SHOULD NOT BE APPLIED** to any recently traumatized neck injury where there is soreness, swelling, or sharp pain present. **Cold therapy** is the appropriate treatment. Heat is most effective in reducing muscle spasms 3-5 days after the initial injury. At this time heat should be applied every two hours for 10-15 minutes and **no more**.

SIMULTANEOUS HEAT AND COLD

When fast results are required, heat and cold therapy are used simultaneously to reduce pain and spasms in muscle tissue.

Cold therapy applied to the region of the muscle spasm, while applying heat to a nearby region of the injury, will relax muscle contractions. As an example, heat on the base of the neck and a cold pack on the mid-back will eliminate the shivering reflex (which can cause further muscle spasms), allowing a speedier recovery from the pain and stress brought about by the injury.

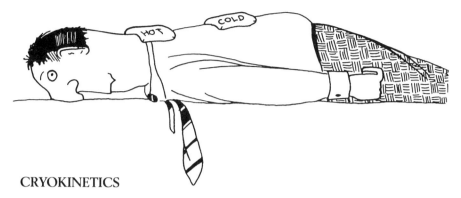

CRYOKINETICS

This is a process using cold therapy while exercising the injured area at the same time.

Cold therapy, which decreases the pain reflex, used in conjunction with exercises accelerates the rehabilitation of the injured area.

22

Neck Posture and Jaw Pain: "Chewing the Fat" Can Be Painful

"Stand tall; don't let your head fall."
S.S. NEEL

Anatomically, the first movable joint encountered closest to the brain is the jaw, which is regulated by the **masseter muscle**. It is this muscle that controls our ability to yawn, grind, chew, and close our mouths. For its size, the **masseter** is the strongest muscle in our body. It is this muscle which when affected by the disease called **tetanus** produces the condition known as **lock jaw** (spasm in this muscle causes a locking of the jaw, or inability to open the mouth).

Most people will at some point in time experience jaw pain. The reasons for jaw pain include an abssessed tooth, grinding of the teeth, chewing gum, or a punch in the jaw! However, the position of the neck may influence the position of the jaw and the degree of force exerted on the **masseter** muscle. For example, if a person is hunched forward – as in the case of an architect poring over design specifications, or a quality control checker – extra pressure is exerted on jaw muscles, causing fatigue, tension, and jaw pain.

TO VERIFY THE EFFECT OF IMPROPER FORWARD NECK POSTURE, PERFORM THE FOLLOWING EXERCISE:

- Sit or stand up straight with your eyes and head level to the ground.
- Touch the palate or the roof of your mouth with your tongue.
- Your teeth should be lightly touching one another but not clenched together.
- In this position the teeth are aligned equally.

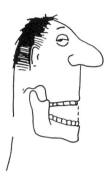

- Gently nod your head forward and you will notice that your upper teeth override the jaw.

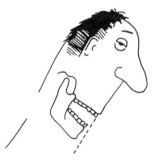

This exercise demonstrates how improper neck posture exerts tension on the jaw muscles, which in turn causes head and neck pain.

When we relax, it is important that we maintain correct upright posture to avoid jaw pain.

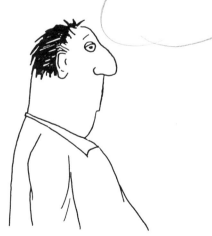

23

Wry Neck: Acute Spasmodic Torticollis

"If only words could describe how I feel."
S.S. NEEL

Wry neck or **torticollis (tor''ti-kol'is)** is an intermittent or continuous painful spasm of the upper back and neck muscles – those known as the **sterno-cleido-mastoid (SCM), scalenus and trapezius** muscle groups.

When the **SCM** muscle group seizes up, the result is a one-sided spasm that causes the patient to turn, tilt or rotate the head in the opposite direction – while flexing the neck to the same side – in an attempt to quell what one patient described vividly as "an excruciating, burning sensation, like hot tar being poured into the muscles of the neck."

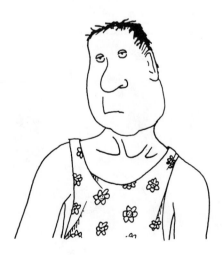

This benign or non-malignant disorder is experienced most frequently by very tense, stressed or anxious individuals. In very rare cases, it is hereditary and called **congenital torticollis.**

Many patients complain they have awakened "to find my neck locked in this position."

In this example, the patients are very stressed or tense, experience nightmares, and have shallow breathing, and their heads would be positioned to one side during sleep. Their bodies (unlike that of a relaxed patient, whose body uses the diaphragm for breathing during sleep) recruit the upper back and neck muscles to "pull up" the lungs to take in oxygen. As this cycle continues the muscles become overworked and fatigued, resulting in the painful spasms of wry neck.

If left untreated, the condition will gradually disappear, usually in 5 to 7 days. Neglect or lack of treatment, however, will complicate wry neck, causing frequent recurrence of the disorder.

TREATMENT AND PREVENTION:

Self-treatment is directed at fatiguing the muscle that spasms by utilizing an **isometric exercise** on the side of the pain or injury. For example:
- If you are experiencing a **wry neck** on the right side, **do not** turn the neck to the left rapidly.
- **Instead**, place the palm of your hand in an upright and supportive manner to the side of your face, on the right side.
- Gently apply an outward pushing motion with your head against the flat of your hand, and at the same time, exert a gentle inward push with your palm.
- **Hold** this contraction for 10 seconds, and release.
- **Carefully** side bend your head in the opposite direction (to the left) as far as you can go until the pain intensifies noticeably on the right-hand side.

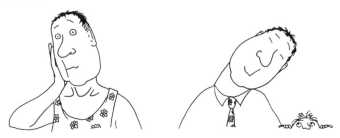

Repeat this procedure 3 times every hour until normal movement is restored and pain abates.

24

Stress, Tension, Emotional Problems and Neck Pain

"Worms eat you when you're dead; worries eat you up when you're alive."

S tress is a physical and emotional reaction to change. It can be either negative or positive, but to the body, stress is stress. Two extreme examples of stress would be:

1. winning a million-dollar lottery
2. having your life savings wiped out overnight

The body's reaction to stress will be the same in both cases: increase in heart rate, tension, and sweating, perhaps with an overproduction of insulin and adrenalin. However, with a million- dollar win at least a person can take a long, languid vacation, pay off all his or her debts and have the potential to be mortgage free.

But the consequences of the grinding cycle of negative or bad stress such as financial worries, family pressures, emotional and work-related problems will eventually take its toll in the form of ill health, "dis-ease" and feeling unable to cope.

Initially, one of the most common symptoms will be a **"pain in the neck."**

The tension and fatigue associated with such a negative cycle causes the upper back and neck muscles to go into "knots." Breathing patterns may become laboured, changing from deep abdominal to shallow rib breathing. Headaches may also occur, ranging from mild discomfort to the blinding pain of excruciating migraines.

TREATMENT AND PREVENTION:

Simple techniques such as stretching and breathing exercises are an excellent starting-place to help you deal effectively with everyday stressors. Information on other techniques such as autogenics, progressive muscle relaxation, creative visualization and bio-feedback can be obtained from your practitioner. However, these techniques should not be used to replace conventional psychotherapy in severe cases.

When dealing with day-to-day stress, it is important to retrain your body to breathe from the diaphragm. To achieve this, practise the following breathing "ratio":

INHALE	HOLD	EXHALE
2 SECONDS	4 SECONDS	3 SECONDS

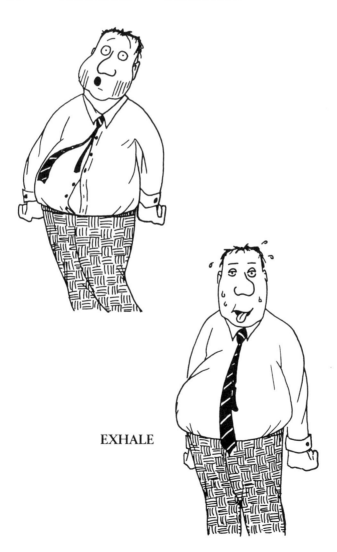

INHALE

EXHALE

Try this daily for 5-10 minutes. You may wish to increase the holding ratio by 2, 3, or 4 seconds, depending on your lung capacity. Remember, the object is to help you deal with stress and to breathe properly, not to stress you by asking you to hold your breath for longer than is comfortable.

The more you practise, the stronger your lungs and their capacity will become, and you will increase the oxygen content of blood circulating to the brain and tissues. The stretching exercises outlined in this book combined with proper breathing will help to reduce the stress-related pain in your neck.

25

Occupational Pain Triggers

*"They intoxicate themselves with work so
they won't see how they really are."*
ALDOUS HUXLEY

The average person's head weighs **10** pounds. To maintain a balance to the head and to correct neck posture, a 10-pound muscular force is exerted by the neck muscles. For every one-inch shift from the head's centre of gravity, the same neck muscles must recruit an additional 10-pound force.

For example, a person employed as an assembly line quality-control checker, who is required to bend over a moving conveyor belt to eyeball products as they pass by, will be in a position where his or her head leans forward 4 inches from the normal centre of gravity. In this case, the muscles supporting the head will require an extra **40**-pound force to do their job – that is, to hold up the head! When this type of activity is pursued over long

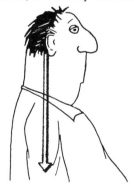

A 10-pound weight is held above the centre of gravity.

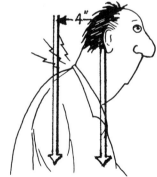

A 4-inch forward shift places approximately 40 pounds of weight on the base of neck.

periods, the body considers this to be an imbalance of what nature intended. The muscles revolt against the undue stress on the ligaments and
joints of the neck. And, as we have discussed earlier, this out-of-alignment
posture may eventually lead to osteoarthritic changes in the neck.

In **Do You Have Good Neck Posture?** (chapter 2) the effects of overall
posture on neck pain were discussed. We are now going to explore how various occupations will affect the integrity of the neck structure.

TYPISTS

Typists who are transcribing from books on their right side will have
their neck turned in a clockwise direction for long periods of time. This
causes a shortening and stiffening of the upper right back and neck muscles,
with subsequent pain in this region.

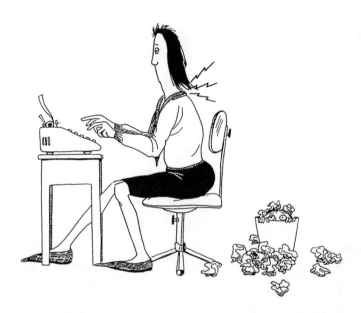

TRUCK DRIVERS

A truck driver has to sit in one position with hands, and arms extended
for long periods, while travelling over rough and bumpy roads. He or she
must use a high degree of concentration with the arms extended, to
maneuver a 24-wheel rig. The driver's somewhat stationary posture, and
prolonged arm and hand extension to grip the wheel place stressors on the
upper back and neck, causing painful tightening of the muscles.

TELEPHONE SOLICITORS

Telephone solicitors habitually crick their necks to one side, to cushion their heads on a telephone neck-and-head-rest or to position the receiver on their shoulder to leave their hands free for writing, order taking, etc. As in the case of the typist and truck driver, muscles stiffen and tighten, with resulting muscle spasm and pain in varying degrees.

CONSTRUCTION WORKERS

It is not unusual for construction workers to flip or torque their necks backward to adjust hard hats that have slipped over their eyes. Over a period of time, this traumatizes the neck. Pain, muscle stiffness and headaches will result.

AUTOMECHANICS

Automechanics spend hours working under car hoists in limited and cramped spaces, with their head and neck extended upward. This posture will "jam" neck joints, and induce spasm in the muscles at the same time, causing a pain syndrome similar to that experienced by the other workers above.

SURGEONS, DENTISTS, MANUAL THERAPISTS

These occupations require long periods of standing and neck flexion. This precipitates muscle fatigue and tightening, which will radiate pain and other symptoms to the head and neck region.

ATHLETES

Boxers and football players are, in a manner of speaking, participants in head-banging sports activities. They are at high risk for injuries, related pain and ongoing symptoms. The cause of their pain is discussed below in **Sports Injuries: Are You a Head Banger?** (chapter 28).

TREATMENT AND PREVENTION:

Occupational treatment and prevention exercises should be done in a reverse direction to the job-related posture or stance. For example, the typist with right-sided pain should stretch the neck to the left side and extend backwards. The automechanic who continually extends the neck upward must exercise the neck by flexing forward.

The procedures outlined in **Exercises For a Healthy Neck** (chapter 32) can easily be modified to suit the occupational requirements of the individual.

26

What Are You Wearing Around Your Neck?

*"There are some on whom fine clothes
weep."*
MONTAIGNE

Have you ever wondered if your headache or neck pain could be attributed to what you are wearing around your neck?

I have treated numerous "white collar" patients complaining of neck and head pain. All of them had been wearing a shirt with an extremely tight collar and a necktie that was tightly knotted. These factors were directly responsible for their symptoms.

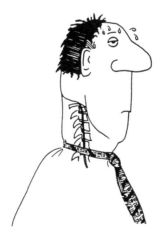

The **carotid artery** is the primary vessel supplying blood from the heart to the head – and is the artery in the neck used by athletes to check their pulse rate during exercise. Because the **carotid artery** is situated just under the skin's surface, a tight collar and knotted tie will easily constrict the blood flow to the head, causing intermittent and restricted flow, and a decrease in oxygenated blood, with resultant headaches.

A camera or binoculars hanging around the neck place undue stress on the back of the neck, causing the base to be pulled forward, resulting in lower neck pain.

Even heavy costume jewelry such as rope pearls, glass beads or heavy gold chains will have a "pulling down" effect, causing discomfort on the back of the neck.

Weighty handbags or purses strapped or straddled across the neck or shoulder will also cause the upper back and neck to be pulled to one side, forcing the muscles in that region to be pushed out of balance.

TREATMENT AND PREVENTION:

The best treatment and prevention would be to have shirt collars that are sized accurately. (A quick check you can do yourself is to place a finger between the collar and the neck – if it's snug, it's probably too tight.) Wear clothes that fit properly, and avoid items around the neck that are associated with the onset of your symptoms.

27

Childbirth and the Child's Neck

*"Children naturally want to be like their
parents and do what they do."*
WILLIAM COBBETT

A s a baby travels through the birth canal, its neck is forced to withstand tremendous pressure. If complications arise during labour, requiring the use of forceps or suction devices, neck stress on the infant child will be intensified.

After the baby is born, its muscles are flimsy and its neck bones are soft and cartilagenous. It is absolutely imperative, therefore, that until the infant starts crawling, the head be cradled and supported to avoid damaging the fragile neck structures.

At the age of two or younger, a child begins actively to explore its environment, tottering about, frequently falling and banging the head and neck. Fortunately, the flexible nature of an infant's bony system allows it to bend rather than break. As tissues are not fully developed and are more flexible, the child can move its neck with greater ease and in more directions than an adult whose movements by comparison are limited, due to hardened and stiffened neck and back muscles. Also, a child's response or recovery time to traumatic injuries is usually only half as long as an adult's.

At the elementary school level, very little emphasis is placed on the importance of correct posture. It is seldom that a child experiences neck pain; as a result, negative postural habits are easily formed. In our society we condition children to floss and brush their teeth regularly, yet pay little attention to the importance of good spinal hygiene. Annual **SPINAL CHECK-UPS** are as important to evaluate the integrity of the control centre of the body as are yearly **physical checkups** that monitor the development of the child.

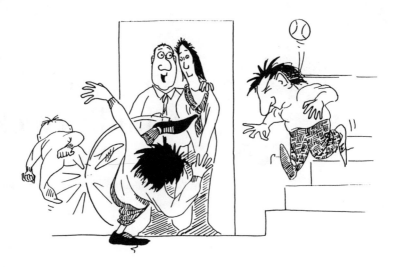

SURE ARE PLAYFUL TODAY, AREN'T THEY?

During puberty, when some teens grow faster than their peers, slouching and drooping their necks in an attempt to be the same height and size as everyone else becomes a habit that is carried over into adulthood. They should gently be encouraged to take pride in their height and to walk upright with a confident manner.

In the absence of significant injuries, correct postural training will guarantee a lifetime free of neck and back pain.

28

Sports Injuries: Are You A Head Banger?

"Pro football is like nuclear warfare. There are no winners, only survivors."
FRANK GIFFORD, *SPORTS ILLUSTRATED*

Football, boxing, ice hockey and wrestling are contact sports recognized as being in a high-risk category for neck injury. And, unlike injuries sustained through car and occupational accidents and muggings, the disabilities sustained through these sports are expected. As a result, athletes train their necks and backs so they can endure excessive and abnormal amounts of force.

To condition the neck, a boxer will spend hours in the gym maintaining a straight posture while sparring with the trainer, who will be rapidly punching and jabbing the head and neck region.

Football players will strengthen their necks by practising one-on-one tackling (going head to head, helmet on, with another player).

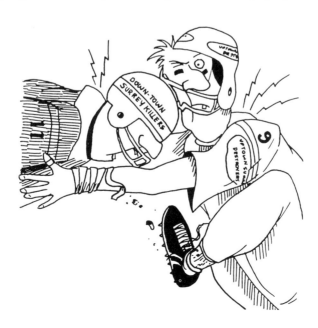

When harm does occur as a result of a sports injury, regardless of the training of the athlete's body, damage is usually severe, with frequent injury to the bony structure as well as to the soft tissues. When the extent of the injury has been verified and diagnosed by way of x-ray examination, surgical intervention may be required.

TREATMENT AND PREVENTION:

The best preventive program is to improve the strength of the neck muscles by exercise; however, nothing will guarantee immunity from injury.

29

Sex and the Neck

"It was worth the pain."
SANDRA CRAIG, WHIPLASH PATIENT

Sexual dysfunction such as impotence, lack of libido and hypersentivity to touch are common complaints of Whiplash patients who have sustained soft tissue injury. Are they merely crying wolf or do they have a legitimate problem?

Certainly the problem cannot be discounted, because in some cases it has jeopardized relationships to the point of separation.

Pain, disability or irritability due to lack of muscle function and spasms all combine to restrict the mobilty of a traumatized body. At times, the simple act of moving the head and neck when kissing can place undue stress on the neck, causing a flare-up of symptoms.

Gentle caressing as in a light touch or a soft massage is also enough to cause pain in a severely traumatized patient. The body tightens up and says, **"Stop – don't touch me!"**

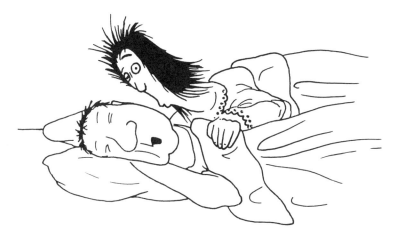

NOT TONIGHT HONEY, I HAD
AN ACCIDENT.

During sexual arousal there is an overall increase in adrenalin production. The heart rate and blood pressure increase, while breathing accelerates. The overall excitement escalates the blood flow to the neck and head, and the patient feels as if the head will explode.

Different body positions can place the head and neck in vulnerable states and cause more damage. The patients in some cases may not be aware of the additional trauma they are precipitating during sexual activity. But afterwords, when they are in a resting mode, the stress caused to the damaged area will be acutely felt, although some may feel it was worth the pain.

In cases of Whiplash injury, the excuse **"Not tonight; I have a headache"** must be given the fullest consideration.

30

The Importance of Feeding Your Neck Tissues Well

"Diet cures more than the lancet."

Pain reduction is a major concern for both the patient and health practitioner. The use of "painkilling" drugs is the most frequent method of treatment, while rehabilitation and therapeutic exercises are the second line of defence in the healing process.

Nutrients are the absolute cornerstone in the making and maintenance of strong, healthy and vibrant body tissues. Yet, the nutritional growth of damaged tissues is the most neglected aspect in healing an injured neck.

The Merck Manual (known as the Medical Bible to many health practitioners) outlines the necessity of the following **micro-nutrients, vitamins and elements** for optimum body functioning:

MICRO-NUTRIENTS	FUNCTIONS
VITAMIN B$_1$ (Thiamine)	Central and peripheral nerve cell function.
VITAMIN B$_2$ (Riboflavin)	Many aspects of energy and protein metabolism.
VITAMIN C (Ascorbic acid)	Essential to bony tissue, collagen formation, tissue respiration and wound healing.
POTASSIUM	Muscle activity, nerve transmission.
CALCIUM	Bone formation, neuromuscular irritability, muscle contractility.
PHOSPHORUS	Energy production.
MAGNESIUM	Nerve conduction, muscle contraction.

A balanced supplementation of these micro-nutrients, recommended by a nutritionally trained health care practitioner, will aid in faster and more effective healing of the damaged neck tissues.

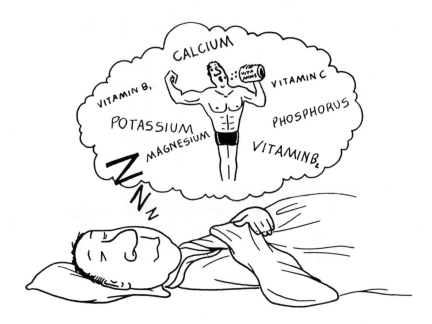

31

Choosing A Practitioner

*"Every physician almost hath his favourite
disease."*
HENRY FIELDING

Professionals in the healing arts agree on the "anatomical" and "physiological" properties of the body: namely, that the normal neck has seven bones and the first bone is called the **atlas**. However, it is at this juncture that the collective agreement ends. For example, examination and treatment of an injured neck by two health practitioners from the same profession frequently results in two different **diagnoses** and methods of treatment.

This problem in diagnosis and treatment is further compounded when a patient seeks advice and help from practitioners in other health care disciplines.

The scope of this book is not to outline all the therapies and treatment modalities available. (This will be dealt with in a future publication.) The focus is to educate the layperson, and to provide self-help exercises which can be safely performed at home and easily monitored by your practitioner.

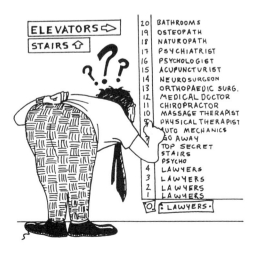

32

Exercises for A Healthy Neck

"There can be no acting or doing of any kind, 'til it be recognized that there is a thing to be done; the thing once recognized, doing in a thousand shapes becomes possible."
THOMAS CARLYLE

The following exercises are designed to prevent disability, to improve impaired function and to increase the optimum level of performance. These therapeutic exercises will assist in correcting postural deviations, aligning the body and stabilizing the joint mechanics.

Incorporate these exercises into your daily routine for a healthy and flexible neck.

EXERCISES FOR INCREASING MOBILITY AND FLEXIBILITY

Do the following exercises slowly and rhythmically.

EXERCISE 1

- Take the neck to the end of movement or to the point of pain.
- Hold the stretch for 10 seconds.
- Repeat 10 times in each direction, as illustrated below.

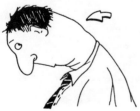

FLEXION

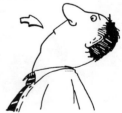

EXTENSION

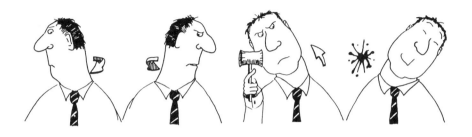

ROTATION   LATERAL BENDING

EXERCISES TO RELEASE TENSION IN THE UPPER BACK AND NECK

In the following exercises, begin by standing tall and drawing or retracting your chin backward into the neck.

EXERCISE 2

- Hold this contraction for 5 seconds; repeat 10 times.

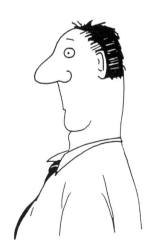

EXERCISE 3

- Stand as above and interlock your hands behind you.
- Draw both your shoulder blades together.
- At the same time, attempt to pull your head up toward the ceiling.
- Hold this contraction for 5 seconds; repeat 10 times.

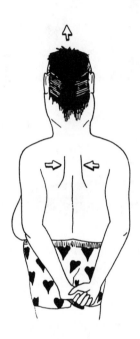

EXERCISE 4

- Stand with your arms hanging down beside you.
- Slowly rotate your shoulders forward in a circular motion, gently increasing the size of the circles. Repeat this 10 times.
- Now reverse the direction of motion and do this also 10 times.

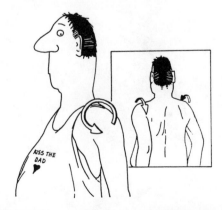

EXERCISE 5

- Stand tall with your arms hanging down beside you.
- Slowly shrug both your shoulders up toward your ears.
- Hold this contraction for 5 seconds; repeat 10 times.

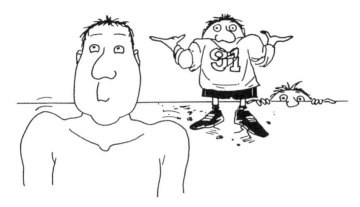

EXERCISE 6

- Stand tall, bend your elbows and bring them to shoulder level (see diagram below).
- Hold this contraction for 5 seconds and repeat 10 times.

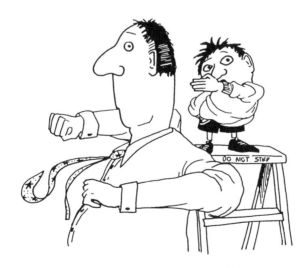

IT'S NICE TO SEE THAT YOU DIDN'T FORGET YOUR ANNIVERSARY, DAD, BUT YOU BETTER PRACTISE A LOT MORE IF YOU WANNA TAKE HER OUT DANCIN!

EXERCISE 7

- Lie on your back and draw your chin in toward your neck.
- Rotate both your shoulders outward and backward.
- Hold this contraction for 5 seconds; repeat 10 times.

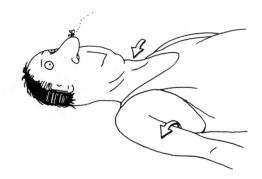

NECK AND UPPER BACK STRENGTHENING ISOMETRIC EXERCISES

Begin all exercises by standing tall with your chin retracted.

EXERCISE 8

- Interlock your hands behind your head, and applying equal pressure, gently push your head into the palms of your hands.
- Hold this contraction for 5 seconds. There should be no movement. Repeat this exercise 10 times.

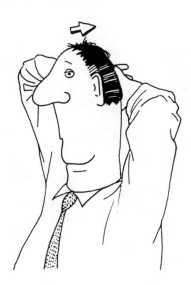

EXERCISE 9

- Interlock your hands over your head. Apply equal pressure upward and downward, with no movement.
- Hold this contraction for 5 seconds; repeat 10 times.

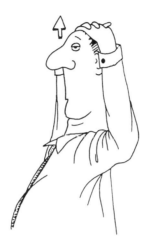

EXERCISE 10

- Interlock your hands in front of your forehead.
- Applying equal pressure, hold the contraction for 5 seconds. Repeat this exercise 10 times.

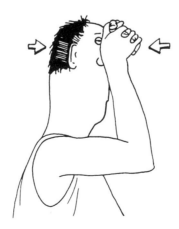

EXERCISE 11

- Bracing the side of the face with your palm, gently apply equal pressure into the palm with your face.
- Hold this contraction for 5 seconds and repeat 10 times.

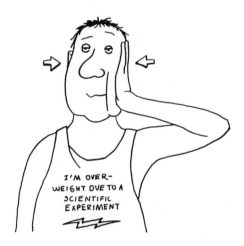

EXERCISE 12
THE 747 EXERCISE

This exercise position mimics the 747 jet. Lie on a mat or carpet with a pillow under your chest so that your face is elevated and centred.

- Begin by placing both your arms extended beside you. **Do not** interlock your hands.
- Slowly draw both your shoulder blades together.
- Simultaneously, gently elevate your face from the ground and retract your chin backward into your neck. Keep your head level with your mid-back. **Do not extend** your head backward, as this may cause **headache** if done incorrectly.
- With shoulder blades drawn together and chin retracted, hold this position for 5 seconds. Repeat 10 times.

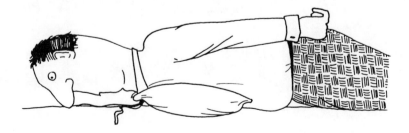

Complete your entire exercise routine by lying on the ground with a pillow supporting the curve of the neck, and rest for 5 minutes. Release any tension by performing breathing exercises.

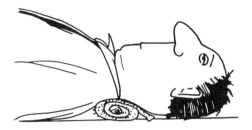

33

Smashing Excuses

"Laughter is the best medicine."

A long list of explanations for automobile accidents are received by insurance companies, such as:

"The pedestrian had no idea which direction to go, so I ran over him."

"The car collided with mine without warning me of its intention."

"I had been driving my car for 40 years when I fell asleep at the wheel and had an accident."

"I pulled over to the side of the road, glanced at my mother-in-law, and headed over the embankment."

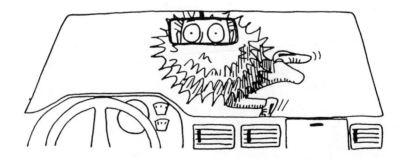

"As I reached the intersection, a hedge sprang up, obscuring my vision."

"The guy was all over the road. I had to swerve a number of times before I hit him."

"I saw an extremely sad-faced man bouncing over the hood on my car."

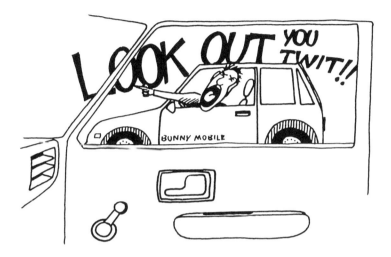

"The indirect cause of the accident was a little guy in a small car with a big mouth."

"I knocked the man over. He admitted it was his fault as he had been knocked over before."

"The car was being used for pleasure purposes – attending the mother-in-law's funeral."

"It is particularly unfortunate that this charge of careless driving has been brought against me, as it is the only thing I can do really well."

"I knew that the dog was possessive about the car, but obviously I would not have asked her to drive if I had thought there was any risk."

"I consider neither vehicle was to blame, but if either was to blame it was the other one."

"The man claimed he and his girlfriend were making love in their small car when another car hit them from behind. The impact momentarily made them lose control, resulting in the pregnancy."

34

Goodbye Pain in the Neck!

"Every day in every way, I am getting better and better."
EMIL COUÉ

Checklist for a healthier neck:

When walking, sitting or standing, make a mental note to check on the position of your chin. It should be retracted or withdrawn, complemented by correct posture: shoulders drawn back, stomach held in. After a while this posture will become a good habit and you will do it automatically.

Keep your head in line with your body – not like the ostrich, jutting forward.

Practise range and motion exercises daily to ensure optimum neck and head mobility:
   - Rotate your head from side to side.
   - Bend your head and neck forward and backward.
   - Side-bend your neck equally on both sides.

When you are stressed or in stressful situations, be mindful of how tension can settle in the neck and upper back muscles. Before stress has a chance to act on your neck, breathe in deeply from the diaphragm and exhale. As you exhale, imagine all your aches and pains exiting at the same time. Proper breathing techniques are also an effective way to rid yourself of a stress-related headache.

Make choosing a pillow that is supportive, the correct height, comfortable and that conforms to **your** neck, a **number one priority!**

If your occupation requires that your neck be maintained in a repetitive or constant position throughout the day, counter-stretch to the opposite side. This simple and unobtrusive action will relieve tension and neck pain.

Wear clothes that fit properly. In particular, clothes should not be too tight, as in a shirt collar or brassiere that is too small and too tightly fitting across the back. Remember that heavy handbags and jewelry around the neck will aggravate healthy soft tissues of the neck and be double trouble for injured soft tissues.

Use cold therapy to assist in healing acute injuries, take appropriate nutritional supplements, and practise **correct** exercise techniques.

If you have osteoarthritis in your neck, do exercise the neck **gently** with the objective of increasing the neck's mobility while decreasing pain. And keep your neck **warm** in damp, cold weather.

There is no greater force than self-motivation. Remember **IT'S YOUR BODY** and **IT'S YOUR HEALTH**. Encourage yourself to get better and work in partnership with your health care practitioner.

Happy Necking!

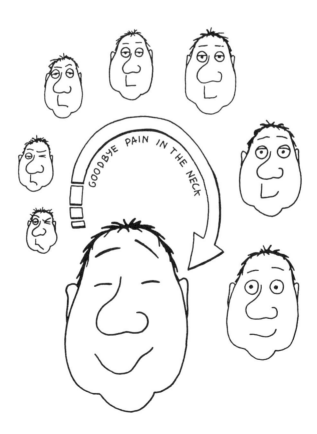

35

Additional Suggested Reading on Neck and Whiplash Injuries

Abel MS, *Radiologic Aspects of Moderately Severe Cervical Spine Trauma*, Arch Phys Med Rehab 40:371, 1959.

Allen WL et al., *Symposium on Whiplash Injuries*, Int Record of Med 169:1-31, 1956.

Ameis A, *Cervical Whiplash: Considerations in the Rehabilitation of Cervical Myofascial Injury*, Can Fam Physician 32:1871-6, September 1986.

Ameis A, Urovitz E, *Whiplash – The Complete Guide to Living With the Pain of Neck Injury*, Toronto: Seal Books, 1988.

Arie ME, *Seat Belt Legislation: Do Patients With Arthritis Need Exemption?* Ann Rheum Dis 41:634, 1982.

Arie ME, Boothroyd F, *Arthritis and Seat Belts*, Lancet p 860, October 8, 1983.

Aubrey JB et al., *Layperson's Knowledge About the Sequelae of Minor Head Injury and Whiplash*, J Neurol Neurosurg Psych 52 (7): 842-6, July 1989.

Backwinkel KD, *Injuries From Seat Belts*, JAMA 205:305-8, 1968.

Bakody J, *Role of the Neck in Head Pain*, Ind Med Surg 19(5):204-6, 1960.

Balla JI, *The Late Whiplash Syndrome*, Aust NZ J Surg 50(6):610-616, 1980.

Balla JI, *The Late Whiplash Syndrome: A Study of an Illness in Australia and Singapore*, Cult Med Psychiatry 6(2):191-210, 1982.

Balla JI, et al., *Whiplash Headache*. Clin Exp Neurol 23:179-82, 1987.

Baron JB, Tangapregasson MJ, Ushio N, Debay A, Bonet J, *Neurotransmitters Dysregulation Related to the Orthostatic Postural Activity Disorders in Case of Post Concussional Syndrome After Head or Whiplash Injuries*, Int J Neurol 12:237-49, 1979.

Baumeister WW, *Chronically Acute Cervical Spine Sprains: A New, Different, Painless and Effective Mode of Manipulation*, Am Chiropractor pp 21, 22, 24, May 1984.

Bayan EE, *The Traumatic Cervical Root Syndrome*, ACA J Chiro 4(4):S25-7, 1967.

Becker RE, *Whiplash Injuries*, In: Barnes MW (ed), Academy of Applied Osteopathy Year Book, Carnel, California: Academy of Applied Osteopathy, 1964:91-5.

Beetham R, *Whiplash Injuries of the Cervical Spine*, Aust J. Physiotherapy 7(3):77-80, 1971.

Bernard, *What the Defense Should Know About Magnetic Resonance Imaging (MRI)*, Personal Injury Law: Defense Bulletin, June 1987.

Beryman JS, *Diagnosis of Whiplash Injuries*, JAMA 152:1698, 1953.

Billing HE, Jr., *The Mechanism of Whiplash Injuries*, International Record of Med and G. P. Clinics pp 2-7, January 1956.

Billing HE, *Traumatic Neck, Head and Eye Syndrome*, J International College of Surgeons pp 558-60, November 1953.

Bilo HJG, Van Vuuren ZC, *Atypical Lumbar Spine Injury from a Two-point Seatbelt*, J Trauma 19(11):841-5, 1979.

Bland J, *Disorders of the Cervical Spine*, W.B. Saunders, 1987.

Blumenthal LS, *Injury to the Cervical Spine as a Cause of Headache*, Postgraduate Med 56(3):147-53, September 1974.

Bocchi L, Osro CA, *Whiplash Injuries of the Cervical Spine*, Italian J Ortho and Trauma 9(Suppl):171-81, 1983.

Braaf MM, Rosner D, *Symptomatology and Treatment of Injuries of the Neck*, New York State J Med 55:237-43, 1955.

Braaf MM, Rosner S, *Meniere-Like Syndrome Following Whiplash Injury of the Neck*, J Trauma 2:494-501, 1962.

Braaf MM, Rosner S, *Whiplash Injury of the Neck – Fact or Fancy?* Int Surg Dig 46:176-82, 1966.

Braunstein P, Moore J, *The Fallacy of the Term Whiplash Injury*, Amer J Surg 97:522-26, 1959.

Brenner, Friedman, Merrit, et al., *Post Traumatic Headache*, Neurosurgery 379, 1944.

Bucholz RW, et al., *Occult Cervical Spine Injuries in Fatal Traffic Accidents*, J Trauma 19(10):768-71, 1979.

Cailliet R, *Subluxations of the Cervical Spine Including the 'Whiplash' Syndrome*, In: Cailliet R, Neck and Arm Pain, Philadelphia: FA Davis Co., 1967: 60-85.

Cameron BM, *A Whiplash Symposium*, Theory Critique Orthopaedics 2:127-9, 1960.

Cammack KV, *Whiplash Injuries to the Neck*, Am J Surg 93:663-6, 1957.

Campbell HE, *Role of the Safety Belt in 19 Autocrashes*, Bull Am Coll Surg 50:155, 1955.

Capistrant TD, *Thoracic Outlet Syndrome in Cervical Strain Injury*, Minn Med 69(1):13-7, 1986.

Carlsson et al., *Neck Injuries in Rear End Car Collisions*, The Quarterly/Journal (IRCOBI), June 1985.

Carpenter S, *Injury of Neck as Cause of Vertebral Artery Thrombosis*, J Neurosurg 18:849, 1961.

Carrick FR, *Cervical Radiculopathy: The Diagnosis and Treatment of Pathomechanics in the Cervical Spine*, J Manipulative and Physiological Therapeutics 6(3): 129-37, September 1983.

Carroll C, et al., *Objective Findings for Diagnosis of 'Whiplash'*, J of Musculoskeletal Med pp 57-76, March 1986.

Chan RC, *Delayed Onset of L'hermitte's Sign Following Head and/or Neck Injuries*, J Neurosurgery 60:609-12, March 1984.

CIBA, *Acute Cervical Spine Injuries*, Clinical Symposia 32:1,1980.

Cintron E, et al., *The Widened Disk Space: A sign of Cervical Hyperextension Injury*, Diagnostic Radiology pp 639-44, December 1981.

Clemens HJ, Burrow K, *Experimental Investigations on Injury Mechanisms of the Cervical Spine at Frontal and Rear-End Vehicle Impacts* (German Translation), Acta Orthop Unfall-Chir 75:116-45, 1972.

Coburn DF, *Vertebral Artery Involvement in Cervical Trauma*, Clin Orthop 24:61-3, 1962.

Colohan DP, *Emergency Management of Cervical Spine Injuries*, Emergency Physician Services, Abbott Laboratories, 1977.

Crowe HE, *Injuries to the Cervical Spine*. Paper presented at the meeting of the Western Orthopaedic Association, San Francisco, 1928.

Deans GT, *Incidence and Duration of Neck Pain Among Patients Injured in a Car Accident*, Br Med J Vol.292, January 1986.

Denis F, *The Three Column Spine and its Significance in the Classification of Acute Thoracolumbar Spinal Injuries*. Spine 8(8), 1983.

DePalma AF, Subin DK, *Study of the Cervical Syndrome*, Clin Orthop 38:135-42, 1965.

Ebbs, Beckly, Hammonds, Teasdale, *Incidents and Duration of Neck Pain Among Patients Injured in Car Accidents*, Br Med J 292:94-5, 1986.

Epstein BS, Epstein JA, Jones MD, *Lap-Sash Three Point Seat-Belt Fractures of the Cervical Spine*, Spine 3:189-93, 1978.

Farbman AA, *Neck Sprain*, JAMA 223:1010-5, 1973.

Farmer JA, Hug PR, Scott HT, *Neck Injury*, Dig Chiropractic Economics pp 40, 44, 45, November-December 1981.

Farmer JA, Hug PR, Scott HT, *"Whiplash": Today's Chiropractor Can Add*

Validity to Your Case, Today's Chiropractic pp 12-4, May-June 1982.

Fielding JW, *Cineroentgenography of the Normal Cervical Spine*, J Bone and Joint Surg 30-A:1280-82, December 1957.

Fielding JW, *Normal and Selected Abnormal Motion of the Cervical Spine from the Second Cervical Vertebra to the Seventh Cervical Vertebra Based on Cineroentgenography*, J Bone and Joint Surg 46-A:1779-81, December 1964.

Fields A, *The Autonomic Nervous System in Whiplash Injuries*, International Record of Med and G. P. Clinics pp 8-10, January 1956.

Fineman S, Borrelli FJ, Rubinstein BM, Epstein H, Jacobson HG, *The Cervical Spine: Transformation of the Normal Lordotic Pattern into a Linear Pattern in the Neutral Posture: A Roentgenographic Demonstration*, J Bone and Joint Surg 45-A:1179-83, September 1963.

Fischer AA, *Clinical Use of Tissue Compliance Meter for Documentation of Soft Tissue Pathology*, Clinical J Pain 3(1):23-30, 1987.

Fish J, Wright RH, *The Seat Belt Syndrome – Does it Exist?* J Trauma 5:746-50, 1965.

Fisher CM, *Concussion Amnesia*, Neurology 16:826-30, 1966.

Fisher CM, *Whiplash Amnesia*, Neurology 32:667-8, 1982.

Fletcher BD, Brogdon BG, *Seat-Belt Fractures of the Spine and Sternum*, JAMA 200:167-8, 1967.

Foreman S, Croft A, *Whiplash Injuries: The Cervical Acceleration/Deceleration Syndrome*, Williams and Wilkins, 1988.

Frankel CJ, *Medico-Legal Aspects of Injuries to the Neck*, JAMA 169:216-23, 1959.

Frazier RG, *Hazards of Health: Effectiveness of Seat Belts in Preventing Motor Vehicle Injuries*, New Eng J Med 264:1254-6, 1961.

Garrett JW, Braunstein PW, *The Seat Belt Syndrome*, J Trauma 2:220-38, 1962.

Gay JR, *Minor Injuries of the Spinal Column Caused by Traffic Accidents*, Canadian Services Med J 12:131-5, 1956.

Gay JR, Abbott KH, *Common Whiplash Injuries of the Neck*, JAMA 152(18):1698-1704, 1953.

Gelber LG, *Medico-Legal Aspects of Whiplash Injuries*, Mississippi Valley Med J 78:215-6, 1956.

Gershon-Cohen J, Glauser F, *Whiplash Fracture of Cervicodorsal Spinous Process*, JAMA 155:560-1, 1954.

Gikas PW, Huelke DE, *Causes of Deaths in Automobile Accidents: Can Seat Belts Really Save Lives?* Michigan Med 63:351-4, 1964.

Gitelman R, Fitz-Ritson D, *Acceleration/Deceleration Injuries (Whiplash)*, ACA J Chiro 17(4):44-7, 1983.

Goff CW, Alden JV, Aldes JH, *Traumatic Cervical Syndrome and Whiplash*, Philadelphia and Montreal:J.B. Lippincott Co., 1964.

Gorman W, *The Alleged Whiplash "Injury,"* Arizona Med pp 411-3, June 1974.

Gorman W, *Whiplash – A Neuropsychiatric Injury*, Arizona Med pp 414-7, June 1974.

Gotten N, *Survey of One Hundred Cases of Whiplash Injury After Settlement of Litigation*, JAMA 162:865-6, 1956.

Greaves C, *Whiplash by Any Other Name*, Med J Aust 1:34, 1980.

Greenawalt MH, *Effects of Trauma Upon the Joints of the Cervical Spine*, Dig Chiropractic Economics pp 43-4, May-June 1985.

Greenfield J, Ilfeld FW, *Acute Cervical Strain: Evaluation and Short Term Prognostic Factors*, Clin Orthop 122:196-220, 1977.

Gulkelberger M, *The Uncomplicated Post-Traumatic Cervical Syndrome*, Scan J Rehab Med 4:150-3, 1972.

Gundrum LK, *Whiplash Injuries to the Ear*, International Record of Med and G. P. Clinics pp 21-5, January 1956.

Guthkelch AN, *Infantile Subdural Haematoma and its Relationship to Whiplash Injuries*, Br Med J 2:430-1, 1971.

Guy JE, *The Whiplash: Tiny Impact, Tremendous Injury*, Ind Med and Surg 37(9):688-91, 1968.

Hadley LA, *Covertebral Articulations and Cervical Foramen Encroachment*, J Bone and Joint Surg 39-A:910-20, 1957.

Hamel HA, Otis EJ, *Acute Traumatic Cervical Syndrome (Whiplash Injury)*, Southern Med J pp 1171-7, November 1962.

Hamilton, *Seat Belt Injuries*, Br Med J 485, 1968.

Harakal JH, *An Osteopathically Integrated Approach to the Whiplash Complex*, JAOA 74(6):59-74, 1975.

Harris JH, *Radiographic Evaluation of Spinal Trauma*, Ortho Clin of North America 17(1):75-86, January 1986.

Harris JH, Jr., *The Radiology of Acute Cervical Spine Trauma*, Baltimore: Williams and Wilkins, 1978.

Hashimoto I, Yoon-Kil T, *The True Sagittal Diameter of the Cervical Spinal Canal and its Diagnostic Significance in Cervical Myelopathy*, J Neurosurg 47:912-6, December 1977.

Hayes P, et al., *Cervical Spine Trauma: A Cause of Vertebral Artery Injury*, Trauma 20(10):904-5, 1980.

Hinoki M, et al., *Neurotological Studies on the Role of the Sympathetic Nervous System in the Formation of Traumatic Vertigo of Cervical Origin*, Acta Otolaryng (Suppl) (Stockh) 330:185-96, 1975.

Hinoki M, et al., *Studies on Ataxia of Lumbar Origin in Cases of Vertigo Due to Whiplash Injury*, Equilibrium Res 3(1):141-52, 1973.

Hirsch SA et al., *Whiplash Syndrome. Fact or Fiction?* Orthop Clin North Am 19 (4):791-5, Oct. 1988.

Hirschfeld AH, Behan RC, *The Accident Process*, JAMA 186:300-6, 1963.

Hodge JR, *The Whiplash Injury: A Discussion of this Phenomenon as a Psychosomatic Illness*, Ohio St Med J 60:762-8, 1964.

Hodge JR, *The Whiplash Neurosis*, Psychosomatics 12(4):245-9, 1971.

Hodgson VR, Lissner HR, Patrick LM, *Response of the Seated Human Cadaver to Acceleration and Jerk With and Without Seat Cushions*, Human Factors pp. 505-523, October 1963.

Hohl M, *Soft Tissue Injuries of the Neck*, Clin Orthop 109:42-9, 1975.

Hohl M, *Soft Tissue Injuries of the Neck in Automobile Accidents, Factors Influencing Prognosis*, J Bone and Joint Surg 56-A:1675-82, December 1974.

Holbourn AHS, *Mechanics of Head Injuries*, Lancet 2:438-41, 1943.

Holding RA, *Osteopathic Thinking in Whiplash Injuries*, Br Osteop J 15(2):131-4, 1983.

Holding RA, *Osteopathic Thinking – Whiplash Injuries*, Part II, Br Osteop J 16(1):46-8, 1984.

Horn SW, *The 'Locked-In' Syndrome Following Chiropractic Manipulation of the Cervical Spine*, Ann Emerg Med 12(10):648-50, 1983.

Horne G, *Neck Sprains After Car Accidents (letter)*, Br. Med J 299(6690):53 July 1989.

Howland WJ, Curry JL, Buffington CB, *Fulcrum Fractures of the Lumbar Spine: Transverse Fracture Induced by Improperly Placed Seat Belt*, JAMA 193:240-1, 1965.

Huelke DF, Kaufer H, *Vertebral Column Injuries and Seat Belts*, J Trauma 15:304-18, 1975.

Huelke DF, Snyder RG, *Seat Belt Injuries: The Need for Accuracy in Reporting of Cases*, J Trauma 15:20-3, 1975.

Huston RL, Sears J, *Effect of Protective Helmet Mass on Head/Neck Dynamics*, Biomechanical Engineering 103:18-23, 1981.

Jackson R, *Crashes Cause Most Neck Pain*, Am Med News December 5, 1966.

Jackson R, *The Positive Findings in Alleged Neck Injuries*, Am J Ortho 6:178-87, 1964.

James OE, Hamel HA, *Whiplash Injuries of the Neck*, Missouri Med 52:423-6, 1955.

Janecki CJ, Lipke JM, *Whiplash Syndrome*, Am Fam Physician 17(4):144-51, 1978.

Jirout J, *The Influence of Postural Factors of the Dynamics of the Cervical Spine: A Comparison of the Reaction of Vertebrae on Lateroflexion in Sitting and in Recumbency*, Neuroradiology 4:239-44, 1972.

Kahane CJ, *An Evaluation of Head Restraints*, Federal Motor Vehicle Safety Standard 22; Tech Rpt, pp 308-27, February 1982.

Kaufer, Herbert, Hayes JT, *Lumbar Fracture-Dislocation, A Study of Twenty-One Cases*, J Bone and Joint Surg 48-A:712-30, June 1966.

Kazarian LE, Hahn JW, Von Gierke HE, *Biomechanics of the Vertebral Column and Internal Organs, Response to Seated Spinal Impact in the Rhesus Monkey*, In: Proceedings Fourteenth Stapp Car Crash Conference, New York: Society of Automotive Engineers, 1970: 121-43.

Keith WS, *'Whiplash': Injury of the 2nd Cervical Ganglion and Nerve*, Can J Neurol Sci 13(2):133-7, 1986.

Kenna CJ, *The Whiplash Syndrome*, Aust Fam Physician 13(4):256, 258, 1984.

Kihlberg JK, *Flexion-Torsion Neck Injury in Rear End Impacts*, Proceedings of 13th Annual Conference of American Association for Automotive Med, October 1969.

Kuch K, Swinson RP, Kirby M, *Brief Communication: Post-Traumatic Stress Disorder After Car Accidents*, Can J Psychiatry 30:426-7, October 1985.

Kulkowski J, Rost WB, *Intra-Abdominal Injury from Safety Belt in Auto Accident*, Arch Surg 73:970-1, 1956.

Leopold RL, Dillon H, *Psychiatric Consideration in Whiplash Injuries of the Neck*, Pa J 63:358-9, 1960.

Lewis RC, Coburn DF, *Vertebral Artery: Its Role in Upper Cervical and Head Pain*, Missouri Med 53:1059-63, 1956.

Lipow EG, *Whiplash Injuries*, Southern Med J 48:1304, 1955.

Lysell E, *Motion in the Cervical Spine: an Experimental Study on Autopsy Specimens*, Gothenburg, pp 3-61, March 1969.

MacNab I, *Acceleration Injuries of the Cervical Spine*, J Bone and Joint Surg 46-A:1797-9, 1964.

MacNab I, *Acceleration-Extension Injuries of the Cervical Spine*, In: Rothman RH, Simeone FA, (eds), The Spine, Philadelphia: W.B. Saunders Co., 1982.

MacNab I, *The Cervical Spine*. Philadelphia: J.P. Lippincott Company, 1983.

MacNab I, *The "Whiplash Syndrome,"* Orthop Clin North America 2(2): pp 389-403, July 1971.

McKeever DC, *The Mechanics of the So-Called Whiplash Injury*, Orthopaedics 2:3-6, 1960.

McKenzie JA, Williams JF, *The Dynamic Behaviour of the Head and Cervical Spine during 'Whiplash'*, J Biomechanics 4(6-A):477-90, 1971.

Maimaris C, *Neck Sprains After Car Accidents*, Br Med J 299(6691):123, 1989.

Marar BC, *The Pattern of Neurological Damage as an Aid to the Diagnosis of the Mechanism in Cervical Spine Injuries*, J Bone and Joint Surg 56A: 1648-54, December 1974.

Marshall LL, *The "Whiplash" Injury*, Med J Aust 2:26-7, 1976.

Martin GM, *Sprain, Strain and Whiplash Injury*, Phys Ther 39:808-13, 1959.

Martinez JL, Garcia DJ, *A Model for Whiplash*, J Biomechanics 1:23-32, 1968.

Mathewson JH, *Dynamics of Car Crashes*, JAMA 152:1698, 1953.

Matias-Guiu J, Buenaventura I, Cervera C, Codina A, *Whiplash Amnesia*, Neurology p 1259, August 1985.

Mealy K, Brennan H, Fenelon GCC, *Early Mobilisation of Acute Whiplash Injuries*, Br Med J 292:656-7, March 8, 1986.

Merskey H, *Psychiatry and the Cervical Pain Syndrome*, Can Med Assn J 130:1119-21, May 1, 1984.

Middleton JM, *Ophthalmic Aspects of Whiplash Injuries*, International Record of Med and G. P. Clinics pp 19-20, January 1956.

Miles KA et al., *The Incidence and Prognostic Significance of Radiological Abnormalities in Soft Tissue Injuries to the Cervical Spine*, Skeletal Radiol 17(7):493-6, 1988.

Morehouse LE, *Body Functions and Controls in Whiplash Injuries*, International Record of Med and G. P. Clinics pp 11-13, January 1956.

Morris F, *Do Head-Restraints Protect the Neck from Whiplash Injuries?* Arch Emerg Med 6(1):17-21.

Morrow J, *Surgical Anatomy of Whiplash Injuries*, International Record of Med and G. P. Clinics pp 14-8, January 1956.

Murone, Ikuo, *The Importance of the Sagittal Diameters of the Cervical Spinal Canal in Relation to Spondylosis and Myelopathy*, J Bone and Joint Surg 56-B:30-6, February 1974.

Murtagh JE, *Patient Health Education: After Your Accident – A Pain in Your Neck*, Aust Fam Physician 10:617, 1981.

Myers A, *Degeneration of Cervical Intervertebral Discs Following Whiplash Injury*, Bull Hosp, Joint Dis pp 74-85, 1953.

Nagel DB, *Whiplash Injuries of the Cervical Spine*, Radiology 69:822-30, 1957.

Nash CL, Jr., *Acute Cervical Soft-Tissue Injury and Late Deformity: A Case Report*, J Bone Joint Surg 61-A:305-7, 1979.

Neel SS, *Whiplash – The Acute Spasmodic Torticollis*, Dig Chiropractic Economics 31(4):122-4, January 1989.

Neel SS, *Whiplash – Was the Head Rotated?* MPI'S Dynamic Chiropractic p 29, June 1, 1989.

Neel SS, *Whiplash: Radiographic Evaluation and Interpretation of the Lateral Cervical Spine,* Dig Chiropractic Economics 32(1):18-20, July 1989.

Neel SS, *Whiplash – Atlanto-Axial Trauma,* MPI'S Dynamic Chiropractic p 34, October 15, 1989.

Neel SS, *Whiplash – Thoracic Implications,* MPI'S Dynamic Chiropractic p 24, January 17, 1990.

Neel SS, Mercer B, Yong G, *The Relationship Between Whiplash Injury and Subsequent Lower Back Complications,* J Chiropractic Research 1(3):86-8, October 1988.

Neuwirth E, *Vertebral Nerve in Posterior Cervical Syndrome* (Correspondence), New York J Med 55:1380, 1955.

Norris SH, Watt I, *The Prognosis of Neck Injuries Resulting from Rear-End Vehicle Collisions,* J Bone and Joint Surg 65-B:608-11, November 1983.

Nygren A, *Injuries to Car Occupants: Some Aspects of the Interior Safety of Cars,* Acta Otolaryngol (Stockh) 395:105, 1984.

Ogilive-Harris DJ, Lloyd GJ, *Personal Injury: A Medico-Legal Guide to the Spine and Limbs,* Toronto: Canada Law Book Inc., 1986.

Ommaya AK, *Damage to Neural and Other Tissues by Whiplash Injury,* Lawyer's Med J 6(4):379-401, 1971.

Ommaya AK, et al., *Subdural Haematoma After Whiplash Injury,* Lancet 2:237-9, 1969.

Ommaya AK, et al., *Whiplash Injury and Brain Damage,* JAMA 204:285-9, 1968.

O'Neill B, Haddon W, Kelley AB, Sorenson W, *Automobile Head Restraint – Frequency of Neck Injury Claims in Relation to the Presence of Head Restraints,* Am J Pub Health 62:399-406, 1972.

Ottomo M, Heimburger RF, *Alternating Horner's Syndrome and Hyperhidrosis Due to Dural Adhesions Following Cervical Spine Cord Injury,* J Neurosurgery 53:97-100, July 1980.

Overton RM, *Restoring a Cervical Curve, Clinical Discussion and Treatment,* J Natl Chiro Assn 32:31-2, 69, 1962.

Palmateer DC, *Greater Occipital-Trigeminal Syndrome,* Clin Chiro (Arch) 2:46-8, 1972.

Pang L, *The Otological Aspects of Whiplash,* Laryngoscope 81:1381-7, 1971.

Parker N, *Accident Litigants and Neurotic Symptoms,* Med J Aust 2:318-22, 1977.

Partyka S, *Whiplash and Other Inertial Force Neck Injuries in Traffic Acci-*

dents, Paper for Mathematical Analysis Division, National Center for Statistics and Analysis, December 1981.

Patrick LM, *Caudocephalad Static and Dynamic Injuries*, Proceedings of the Fifth Stapp Automotive Crash and Field Demonstration Conf, University of Minnesota, 1962.

Pedigo M, Neel S, Nunno L, Huddleston L, *Whiplash – A Chiropractic Approach to Treatment and Self Care*, Krames Communications, Daly City, California, December 1988.

Pennie BH, *Whiplash Injuries: A Trial of Early Management*, J Bone and Joint Surg 72(2):277-19, March 1990.

Phyllis FA, *Motor Vehicle Occupant Injuries in Noncrash Events*, Place: American Academy of Pediatrics, 838-40, 1980.

Rechtman AM, Borden AG, Gershon-Cohen J, *The Lordotic Curve of the Cervical Spine*, Clin Orthop 20:208, 1961.

Reynolds GG, Pavot AP, Kenrick MM, *Electromyographic Evaluation of Patients With Posttraumatic Cervical Pain*, Arch Physical Med and Rehabil pp 170-3, March 1968.

Richman, *Whiplash: Truly a Pain in the Neck*, The Advocate Delaware Trial Lawyers' Assn, August-October 1988.

Rimel RW, Giordani B, Barth JT, Boll TJ, Jane JA, *Disability Caused by Minor Head Injury*, Neurosurgery 9(3):221-8, September 1981.

Rinehart RE, *Whiplash: Practical Considerations*, Medical Trial Technique Quarterly 28:288-300, 1981.

Roaf R, *A Study of the Mechanics of Spinal Injuries*, J Bone Joint and Surg 42-B:810-23, November 1960.

Robinson GK, *Cinefluoroscopic Motion Studies of the Post Traumatic Cervical Spine*, Dig Chiropractic Economics pp 156-7, November 1984.

Roca PD, *Ocular Manifestations of Whiplash Injuries*, Ann Ophthalmology 4(1):63-73, January 1972.

Roydhouse RH, *Has the Safety-Belt Replaced the Hangman's Noose*, Lancet 8441:1341, June 8, 1985.

Roydhouse RH, *Torquing of Neck and Jaw due to Belt Restraint in Whiplash-Type Accidents*, Lancet 8441:1341, June 8, 1985.

Roydhouse RH, *Whiplash and Temporomandibular Dysfunction*, Lancet pp 1394-5, June 16, 1973.

Rubin D, *Head, Neck and Arm Symptoms Subsequent to Neck Injuries*, Arch Phys Med Rehabil 40:387-9, 1959.

Rubin W, *Whiplash With Vestibular Involvement*, Arch Otolaryngol Vol. 97, January 1973.

Rutherford WH, Greenfield AA, Hayes HRM, Nelson JK, *The Medical Effects of Seat Belt Legislation in the United Kingdom*, London: HMSO, 1985.

Sano K, Nakamura N, *Correlative Studies of Dynamics and Pathology in Whiplash and Head Injuries*, Scand J Rehabil Med 4:47-54, 1972.

Schneider K et al., *Modelling of Jaw-Head-Neck Dynamics During Whiplash*, J Dent Res 68(9):1360-5, September 1989.

Schneider RC, Cherry GL, Pantck HE, *The Syndrome of Acute Central Cervical Spinal Cord Injury*, J Neurosurg 11:546-51, 1954.

Schneider RC, et al., *Lap Seat Belt Injuries: The Treatment of the Fortunate Survivor*, Michigan Med 67:171-86, 1968.

Schneider RC, Schemm GW, *Vertebral Artery Insufficiency in Acute and Chronic Spinal Trauma*, J Neurosurg 18:348, 1961.

Schutt CH, Dohan FC, *Neck Injuries to Women in Auto Accidents: A Metropolitan Plague*, JAMA 206:2689-94, 1968.

Seat Belts Reviewed, Lancet pp 75-6, January 11, 1986.

Selecki BR, *Whiplash: A Specialist's View*, Aust Fam Physician 13(4):243, 246, 247, 1984.

Seletz E, *Whiplash Injuries*, JAMA 168:1750-4, 1958.

Seletz E, *Neurologic Surgery, Trauma and the Cervical Portion of the Spine*, J International College of Surgeons 40(1):47-62, 1963.

Severy DM, *Automobile Crash Effects*, Paper presented before the Engineering Section, California Traffic Safety Conference, Sacramento, California, October 7, 1954.

Severy DM, Mathewson JH, *Automobile Barrier Impacts*, Highway Research Board Bull 91:39, 1954.

Severy DM, Mathewson JH, Bechtol CP, *Controlled Automobile Rear-End Collisions: An Investigation of Related Engineering and Medical Phenomenon*, Can Services Med J pp 727-59, November 1955.

Shkrum MJ et al., *Upper Cervical Trauma in Motor Vehicle Collisions*, J Forensic Scie 34(2):381-90, March 1989.

Simmons EH, *Ulnar Nerve Neuritis Associated with Whiplash Injuries*, Paper given at the meeting of the Canadian Orthopaedic Association, Hamilton, Canada, 1969.

Smith WS, Kaufer H, *A New Pattern of Spine Injury Associated with Lap-Type Seatbelts: A Preliminary Report*, Univ Mich Med Cent J, 33:99-104, 1967.

Smith WS, Kaufer H, *Patterns and Mechanisms of Lumbar Injuries Associated with Lap Type Seat Belts*, J Bone and Joint Surg 51-A:239-54, March 1969.

Snyder R, *Automotive Belt Systems Hazardous to Children?* Am J Dis Child 129:946, 1975.

States JD, Korn MW, Masengill JB, *The Enigma of Whiplash Injuries*, NY State J Med 70(24):2971-8, 1970.

Steckler RM, Epstein JA, Epstein BS, *Seat Belt Trauma to the Lumbar Spine:*

An Unusual Manifestation of the Seat Belt Syndrome, J Trauma 9(6):508-12, 1969.

Stringer WL, et al., *Hyperextension Injury of the Cervical Spine with Esophageal Perforation*, J Neurosurgery 53:541-3, October 1980.

Sube J, Ziperman HH, McIver WJ, *Seat Belt Trauma to the Abdomen*, A J Surg 113:346-50, 1967.

Sunderland S, *Mechanisms of Cervical Nerve Root Avulsion Injuries of the Neck and Shoulder*, J Neurosurgery 41:705-14, 1974.

Syverson OA, *The Neurovascular Syndrome in Whiplash Injuries*, J Natl Chiro Assn 30(11):15-8, 70-3, 1960.

Taillard W, et al., *Orthopaedic Treatment of Whiplash Injuries of the Cervical Spine*, Radiol Clin 44:236-50, 1975.

Tarantino JA, Oliveira DS, *Litigating Neck and Back Injuries*, Santa Ana, California: James Publishing Group, 1989.

Taylor AR, *The Mechanism of Injury to the Spinal Cord in the Neck Without Damage to the Vertebral Column*, J Bone and Joint Surg 33B, November 1951.

Thiemeyer JS, Duncan GA, Hollins GG, *Whiplash Injuries of the Cervical Spine*, Virginia Med Monthly 85:171-4, 1958.

Thomas C, Faverjon G, Hartemann F, Tattiere C, Patel A, Got C, *The Enigma of Whiplash Injuries*, In: Proceedings of the 13th Conference of the American Association of Automative Medicine, 1969, Michigan: Highway Safety Research Unit of University of Michigan, 1970:83-108.

Threadgill FD, *Whiplash Injury – End Results in 88 Cases*, Med Ann DC 20:266-8.

Tourin B, Garrett JW, *A Report on Safety to the California Legislature*, Automotive Crash Injury Research of Cornell University, February 1960.

Tourin B, Garrett JW, *Safety Belt Effectiveness in Rural California Automobile Accidents*, Automotive Crash Injury Research of Cornell University, New York, February 1960.

Ushio N, Hinoki S, Okada S, Ishida Y, Koike S, Shizuku S, *Studies on Ataxia of Lumbar Origin in Cases of Vertigo Due to Whiplash Injury*, Aggressologie 14-D:73-82, 1973.

Von Bahr V, Eriksson E, *Injuries Due to the Use of Safety Belts*, Svensk Lakartidn 58:141-3, 1961.

Vulcan AP, King AI, *Forces and Moments Sustained by the Lower Vertebral Column of a Seated Human During Seat-to-Head Acceleration*, Am Soc Mechanical Engineers pp 84-100, 1970.

Wagner RE, Abel MS, *Small Element Lesions of the Cervical Spine Due to Trauma*, Clin Orthop 16:215, 1960.

Walker JA, *Holiday Drinking and Highway Fatalities*, JAMA 206:2693, 1968.

Walker JI, *Post-Traumatic Stress Disorder After Car Accident*, Postgraduate Med 69(2):82-6, 1981.

Ware M, *Conservative Treatment of Intervertebral Disk Lesions and 'Whiplash' Injury (Editorial)*, Med J Aust 2:30-1, 1975.

Webb MN, Terrett AG, *Whiplash: Mechanisms and Patterns of Tissue Injury*, J Aust Chiropractors' Assn 15(2):60-9, June 1985.

Weinberger LM, *Trauma or Treatment: The Role of Intermittent Traction in the Treatment of Cervical Soft Tissue Injuries*, J Trauma 16(5):377-82, May 1976.

Weir D, *Roentgenographic Signs of Cervical Injury*, Clin Orth and Related Res 109:9-16, June 1975.

Weisner H, Mumenthaler M, *Whiplash Injuries of the Cervical Spine: A Catamnestic Study*, Arch Orthop Unfall-Chir 81:13-36, 1975.

Whitley, Forsyth, *The Classification of Cervical Spinal Injuries*, 83 Am J Roentgenology 83:633, 1960.

Wickstom, *Effects of a Whiplash Injury*, JAMA 194:40, 1965.

Wickstom, La Toca, *Trauma: Head and Neck Injuries from Acceleration/Deceleration Forces*, In: Ruge, Wilste (eds) Spinal Disorders: Diagnosis and Treatment, 1977.

Wiesel SW, Feffer HL, Rothman RH, *Neck Pain*, Virginia: The Michie Co. 1986.

Williams A, Zador P, *Injuries to Children in Automobiles in Relation to Seating Location and Restraint Use*, Accid Annal Prev 9:69, 1977.

Williams JS, Lies BA, Hale HW, *The Automotive Safety Belt: In Saving a Life May Produce Intra-Abdominal Injuries*, J Trauma 6:303-15, 1966.

Williams JW, Kirkpatrick JR, *The Nature of Seatbelt Injuries*, J Trauma 11:207-18, 1971.

Winston KR, *Whiplash and its Relationship to Migraine*, Headache 27(8):452-7, September 1987.

Yarnell PR et al., *Minor Whiplash Head Injury with Major Debilitation*, Brain Inj 2(3):255-8, July-September 1988.

Zatzkin HR, Kveton FW, *Evaluation of the Cervical Spine in Whiplash Injuries*, Radiology 75:577, 1960.

Quotations from unknown sources in the beginning of each chapter have been taken from:

Leo Rosten's Treasury of Jewish Quotations, McGraw Hill, New York, 1972.

The HomeBook of Quotations – Classical and Modern, 10th Edition, Dodd, Mead and Co. New York, 1967.

NOTES:

ORDER FORM

If you cannot obtain a copy of this book from a bookstore, you may use this order form.

Book price per copy **$14.95**. Add postage and handling: $2.00 for the first book, $.75 for each additional book.

Please send me _____ copies of **TREATING NECK PROBLEMS THE NATURAL WAY: GOODBYE PAIN IN THE NECK.**

Total amount enclosed **$** _____

Send to: (Please print)

Dr./Mr./Mrs./Ms. _____

Address _____

City _____

Province/State _____Postal Code/Zip _____

Telephone: Business _____ Home _____

METHOD OF PAYMENT:

_____ Cheque enclosed
_____ Money Order
_____ Visa
_____ MasterCard
Credit Card # _____Expiry Date _____

Signature _____

You can also order by calling (604) 599-8688
FAX your order to (604) 599-5523

Make cheques payable and mail to:
Health Challenges Today Inc.
11133 Prospect Drive
Delta, B.C.
Canada
V4E 2R4